RESEXUALISING LATER LIFE

Sex and Intimacy in Later Life

Series Editors: **Paul Simpson**, University of Manchester,
Paul Reynolds, The Open University and
Trish Hafford-Letchfield, University of Strathclyde

This internationally focused series builds on, extends and deepens knowledge of sexual practice amongst older people. Compiling work by established and emerging scholars across a range of disciplines, it covers the experiential, empirical and theoretical landscapes of sex and ageing.

Also available in the series

Later Life, Sex and Intimacy in the Majority World,
edited by **Krystal Nandini Ghisyawan**, **Debra A. Harley**, **Shanon Shah** and **Paul Simpson**

HIV, Sex and Sexuality in Later Life,
edited by **Mark Henrickson**, **Casey Charles**, **Shiv Ganesh**, **Sulaimon Giwa**, **Kan Diana Kwok** and **Tetyana Semigina**

Desexualisation in Later Life,
edited by **Paul Simpson**, **Paul Reynolds** and **Trish Hafford-Letchfield**

Sex and Diversity in Later Life,
edited by **Trish Hafford-Letchfield**, **Paul Simpson** and **Paul Reynolds**

Find out more at:
policy.bristoluniversitypress.co.uk/sex-and-intimacy-in-later-life

RESEXUALISING LATER LIFE

Performances of Older Sexual Citizenship

Edited by
Paul Reynolds, Paul Simpson and
Trish Hafford-Letchfield

With a foreword by
Raffaella Ferrero Camoletto

First published in Great Britain in 2025 by

Policy Press, an imprint of
Bristol University Press
University of Bristol
1-9 Old Park Hill
Bristol
BS2 8BB
UK
t: +44 (0)117 374 6645
e: bup-info@bristol.ac.uk

Details of international sales and distribution partners are available at policy.bristoluniversitypress.co.uk

British Library Cataloguing in Publication Data
A catalogue record for this book is available from the British Library

ISBN 978-1-4473-6619-5 hardcover
ISBN 978-1-4473-6621-8 ePub
ISBN 978-1-4473-6622-5 ePdf

Cover design: Robin Hawes
Front cover image: Getty/4FR
Bristol University Press and Policy Press use environmentally responsible print partners.
Printed and bound in Great Britain by CPI Group (UK) Ltd, Croydon, CR0 4YY

FSC
www.fsc.org
MIX
Paper | Supporting responsible forestry
FSC® C013604

Bristol University Press's authorised representative in the European Union is:
Easy Access System Europe, Mustamäe tee 50, 10621 Tallinn, Estonia,
Email: gpsr.requests@easproject.com

Contents

Notes on editors and contributors

Editors

Paul Reynolds has taught across northern British universities for over 30 years, attaining the position of Reader in Sociology and Social Philosophy. He currently tutors Open University (UK) courses and provides consultancy on social research approaches and research ethics. His research interests include sexual ethics and literacy, kink and the construction of perversion, Marxism, sexuality, subjectivity and collectivities, and the role and responsibilities of intellectuals.

Paul Simpson has lectured at the University of Manchester and, while 'retired' from full-time paid work, writes and publishes on ageing sexualities. He has published extensively on older gay men, gay male cultures of ageing and, more recently, (in this same series) on later life sex and intimacy in the global South and East. He has more than 50 peer-reviewed publications and has been published in prestigious academic journals such as *Ageing & Society*, *The British Journal of Sociology*, *Men and Masculinities*, *Sociological Research Online*, *Sociological Review*, *Sociology of Health and Illness*, and *The Journal of Sex Research*.

Trish Hafford-Letchfield is Professor of Social Work and Social Policy and ex-Head of School at the University of Strathclyde. Trish is a qualified nurse and social worker. Her research interests include the participatory research experiences of marginalised groups in care contexts for older people, sexuality and gender identity in social work and social care, suicide in later life, leadership, management and organisational development in public services, art-based pedagogies and pedagogies concerning professional care practice. Trish has more than 150 publications on topics relating to care and care services.

Contributors

Liat Ayalon is Professor in the School of Social Work, at Bar Ilan University, Israel. Professor Ayalon is currently funded by the Israel Science Foundation to study intergenerational relations in the context of climate change. She is also funded by the Volkswagen Foundation in collaboration with colleagues in Germany (Dr von Kutzleben and Professor Schweda) to study moral dilemmas in migrant home care arrangements. Also, she was the coordinator of an international EU-funded PhD programme on the topic of ageism (EuroAgeism.eu; 2017–22). Between 2014 and 2018, she has led an international research network on the topic of ageism, funded through COST (Cooperation in Science and Technology; COST IS1402, notoageism.com). She consults both national and international organisations concerning the development and evaluation of programmes and services for older adults. In recognition of her work, Professor Ayalon was selected by the UN Decade of Healthy Ageing as one of 50 world leaders working to transform the world to be a better place in which to grow older.

Christine Beasley is the founder of the Fay Gale Centre for Research on Gender, at the University of Adelaide. She is a Fellow of the Academy of the Social Sciences in Australia. Her recent books include *Living Legacies of Social Injustice: Power, Time and Social Change* (edited with Pam Papadelos, 2023), *Internet Dating: Intimacy and Social Change* (with Mary Holmes, 2021) and *The Cultural Politics of Popular Hollywood Film: Power, Culture and Society* (with Heather Brook, 2019).

Eir-Anne Edgar is Associate Professor of Literature in English at the Norwegian University of Science and Technology (NTNU) in Trondheim, Norway. She writes about race, sexuality and gender in 20th- and 21st-century literature and media. Her work can be found in *Journal of Popular Culture*, *European Journal of American Studies*, *Sexuality & Culture*, and other publications.

Ateret Gewirtz-Meydan is Associate Professor at the University of Haifa's School of Social Work. She specialises in sexual health among older adults, child sexual abuse, and trauma-related sexuality. A certified sex therapist and social worker, she has published in journals such as the *Journal of Sex Research*, *Archives of Sexual Behavior*, and the *Journal of Sexual Medicine*.

Susan Gillen has a Master's degree by research in Sociology and has been lecturing in the social sciences and in the field of health and social care for over 20 years, and is currently working for Edge Hill University, Lancashire. She is also working as a self-employed specialist dementia trainer in the social care sector. Susan has a varied employment background: in addition to her experience of teaching/training adults in a variety of settings including higher education, further education, workplaces and prisons, she has specialist knowledge in the areas of housing and dementia. She also has significant expertise in various issues affecting older people, which has been gained from academic study and employment in the voluntary sector. Besides her focus on older people, Susan's research interests include ageing across the life course, dementia, health inequalities, and identity and place. Her Master's degree thesis, based on qualitative methods, focused on the impact of care workers' constructions of the sexuality of older people resident in care homes, which was motivated by concern about the impact of stereotypes on citizenship status.

Mary Holmes is Professor of Emotions and Society in the Sociology Department at the University of Edinburgh. Her latest books are *Internet Dating: Intimacy and Social Change* (with Christine Beasley) and *Young Refugees and Forced Displacement: Navigating Everyday Life in Beirut* (with Lili Riga et al).

Nathalie Huitema is an adjunct lecturer in the Human Sexuality Department at the California Institute of Integral Studies (CIIS) in San Francisco, an AASECT-certified sex educator, and a registered clinical sexologist in the US. She holds a PhD in Human Sexuality, with a focus on ageing and consent, and worked as a psychologist in Dutch nursing homes for over 15 years. She has developed a range of training programmes on sexuality, ageing and long-term care; presented at national and international conferences; and authored journal articles and book chapters in the field.

Ricardo Iacub has a PhD in psychology and is Professor of Psychology of Ageing at the University of Buenos Aires, Argentina. He teaches various courses relating to narrative and critical gerontology and has published extensively on the subjects of identity, empowerment and erotics in later life.

Barbara L. Marshall is Emerita Professor of Sociology at Trent University, Peterborough, Canada. She has written widely on feminist theory, ageing and the body, and, with colleague Stephen Katz, has co-authored a series of papers exploring ageing, embodiment, sexuality and technologies. Her most recent book is a co-edited collection, *Socio-Gerontechnology: Interdisciplinary Critical Studies of Ageing and Technology* (with A. Peine, W. Martin and L. Neven, Routledge 2021). She continues to research and write while enjoying retirement on the west coast of Canada. Current work draws on several collaborative projects exploring ageing bodies and socio-technical imaginaries of ageing futures.

Tineke Roelofs works as a health care psychologist (currently training as a clinical neuropsychologist) in a specialised Dutch nursing home. As a senior researcher at TRANZO (centre for the study of care and wellbeing, Tilburg University), she supervises PhD students on themes related to ethical dilemmas in nursing homes. She lectures on 'sexuality in the elderly' in the Clinical Psychology Master's programme and is a guest speaker at national (Dutch) and international conferences.

Megan Todd is Senior Lecturer and Course Leader in Social Science at the University of Central Lancashire. She has been involved in a range of research projects, including a UKRI-funded project on the online abuse experienced by minority groups. Her research focuses on sexualities, gender and violence, and she has published extensively on issues relating to gender, feminism, intimacies and sexualities.

Feliciano Villar has a PhD in psychology and is Professor in the Department of Cognition, Development and Educational Psychology at the University of Barcelona. He directs the Master's degree programme in Psychogerontology and coordinates the Research Group on Gerontology. He is interested in the implementation of person-centred care in long-term residential settings and in the policies and practices concerning opportunities for resident social participation and rights, and particularly for people with dementia. Feliciano has published extensively on sex and intimacy in later life care settings, using qualitative, quantitative and mixed research methods, and often as lead author in a research team. More recently, he has published in academic journals such as *Dementia, The European Journal of Ageing, Sexuality Research and Social Policy*, and *The Journal of Advanced Nursing*.

Acknowledgements

We would like to thank the contributors whose critical scholarship, collegiality, hard work and patience have made this volume possible. Paul Reynolds would like to thank J.S., A.L.W., J.B., L.C., A.M., B.B., P.V. and S.G. for their continued support in a less than easy time. Paul Simpson would like to thank his husband, Gordon Blows, and sociology colleagues at the University of Manchester, for many, many fascinating conversations and intellectual and emotional support. Trish Hafford-Letchfield would like to dedicate this book to Aili, Teddy and Nora Letchfield, her three grandchildren, who bring joy to the world.

Series editors' introduction

Paul Reynolds, Paul Simpson and Trish Hafford-Letchfield

This *Sex and Intimacy in Later Life* book series will explore, interrogate and enlighten upon the sensual, sexual and intimate lives of older people. The motivation for launching this series was a concern with the relative lack of attention in public, professional and academic/intellectual spheres to sex and intimacy in later life (indicatively, Hafford-Letchfield, 2008; Simpson et al, 2018a, 2018b). The series is intended to contribute to and enrich the development of the field of studies in the intersections of age, sex, sexuality and intimacy as a critical and important area of scholarship. It is only beginning to be recognised as an important social, cultural and political issue within and beyond the 'Western' academy, from which it has emerged. Its earliest contributions, of which this volume is a part, are motivated by a desire to recognise and reject the pathologies and prejudices that have infused this intersection – what Simpson has termed 'ageist erotophobia' (Simpson et al, 2018b, p 1479) – and fuels the failure to acknowledge older people as sexual agents. This is both an intellectual and a political agenda, to question and evaluate the impact of real rather than assumed losses of cognitive, physical, social and sexual capacity, and to recuperate older people as sexual agents from dismissal, ridicule and trivialisation.

If the latter half of the twentieth century was characterised by challenges to the pathologies of social identities – particularly gender, ethnicity and race, disability, sexuality – and struggles for recognition, rights and liberties, more intersectional struggles and recognitions characterise the twenty-first century (on intersectionality, see indicatively Hancock, 2016; Hill Collins and Bilge, 2016). Significant among these has been the re-evaluation of what it is to age and to be an older agent in contemporary societies. Older people have historically experienced both veneration and respect and neglect and pathology, largely based on differing cultural stereotypes of the value of age (Ylanne, 2012). The most common characterisation is that older people are not sexual, past being sexual or represent a problematic sexuality – or their sexuality is a superficial concern and secondary to concerns of health, care, life course and support by public services and engagement and pensions/resources. Such concerns are those mainly of 'Western' cultures and reflected in the Western influence across the globe in respect of state intervention and provision, but elsewhere they have been subsumed and often rendered invisible into family and kinship structures. Older people's intimate and sexual lives and experiences have transformed in the last 40 years, as a consequence of a number of significant social changes: new technologies – digital, mechanical and pharmaceutical – and their interventions; the recognition of older people as exploitable markets for consumption; healthier lifestyles, changes and extensions to life course and life expectancy; the erosion of social and sexual pathologies around age and recognitions of different intersections and their importance (LGBTQI older people, older people of different ethnicities, older disabled/neurodiverse and 'able-bodied/minded' people, older men and women).[1] These transformations demonstrate evidence of increase in the sexual relations and intimacies of older people and their impacts, such as increased rates of STD transmission, or implications for healthy sex lives for older people in care institutions (indicatively, Drench and Losee, 1996; Lindau et al, 2007; Bodley-Tickell et al, 2008; Chao et al, 2011; Simpson, 2015; Age UK, 2019). The scholarship exploring these developments has only recently begun to catch up. A small but growing literature has focused on age and sexuality (represented in the sources authors draw from in this series), with a principal focus on the erosion of easy pathologies and stereotypes of older people's heteronormativity and heterosexuality.

Particularly as the 'baby boomers' of the 1950s and 1960s move into old age, changed sexual attitudes, wants and needs require changed political, cultural and institutional responses. The older generation of baby boomers in the late 1940s and 1950s may have remembered Vera Lynn (an iconic British wartime singer singing patriotic songs during World War 2) and post-war society – retaining traditional stereotypes of older people. However, their horizons will have been formed and broadened more by influences from the 1960s' pop and rock culture (notably with such artists as the Beatles, Rolling Stones and Janis Joplin), women's and LGBT liberation struggles, the proliferation of accessible public representations of sex and the 'pornification' of society in the digital age.

Ageing and becoming 'older', intimacy, sexual identity, relations and practices, and sexual pleasure are all contested concepts and subject categories. They are understood as being constituted by different demarcations, distinctions and understandings arising from different intellectual disciplines, conceptual approaches, cultures, geographical contexts and historical contexts. While it is neither desirable nor credible to preclude critical and constructive debate on the meanings and demarcations of these intersections, it is necessary to draw some broad conceptual boundaries rather than hard-and-fast definitions.

'Ageing' and 'older' are broad categories that are attached to people considered in their 'third age' or 'later life' – in more affluent countries/regions of the mainly Global North, the threshold is often seen as the age of 50+. This reflects common practice in the literatures of social gerontology, psychology and the sociology of ageing (see Zaninotto et al, 2009; Cronin and King, 2010; Stenner et al, 2011). It is after that, and into their sixth decade, that older people experience a process of de-eroticisation that could be called 'compulsory non-sexuality' (taking our cue from feminist theorist Adrienne Rich (1981), who articulated pressures on women's sexuality towards 'compulsory heterosexuality').

Ageing and being older can be understood mainly in two ways. First, the terms describe ageing as a chronological and physiological process involving key changes, which become particularly marked (and can be stigmatised) in the later stages of the life course. This raises questions around the differential impact of life course experience and physiological change – which may include loss and/or reduction of physical and mental capacities for some people at different stages in the life course. It is structured both by physiological change and by the (often imperceptible) internalisation and normalisation of orthodoxies describing ageing and being older in cultural and social discourse, and everyday practice and experience of how older people are perceived and how older people see themselves – often as lacking – and in relation to younger people (Foucault, 1977, 1978). Such is the means by which older people (as much as younger people or social and cultural institutions) both produce and accept the discursive limits to ageing. Second, ageing and being older could be described as an attribution constituted by ideology and discourse, structural-hierarchical and cultural-discursive influences and material contexts, such as the structure of organisations, public spaces, cultural representations and spaces of connection (for example, labour markets). Ageing is usefully regarded as a product of intersections between the symbolic/discursive and structural/material dimensions of existence. The attribution of a particular age – young, mature or older – is an ideological construct suffused by power relations and composed of cultural attributions, instantiated in material processes and practices. These structural factors impose all manner of constraints on older people's sexual agency (though these can be questioned, challenged and resisted). Put simply, age is a social, cultural and political construct and how older people are perceived and valued – whether prejudicially or with respect – is constituted in the wider character of social values and dominant discourses. While age is an experienced and embodied phenomenon, its meaning is socially, culturally and politically mediated.

'Sex' and 'sexuality' are often distinguished by the former being focused on practices and behaviour, and the latter being focused on identities, relations and orientations. The terms are nevertheless porous and intertwined (Weeks, 2010). Sexuality describes the processes of being sexual (or not) in the world and through self-recognition, expressing (or not) sexual choices and preferences and enjoying (or not) sexual pleasures. It involves the expression of emotions, desires, beliefs, self-presentation and how we relate to others. It most commonly relates to sexual identity – for example hetero, lesbian, gay, bisexual, queer, asexual (Rahman and Jackson, 2010). Sexuality is multidimensional, being co-constituted by the biological (for example bodily sensations interpreted as 'sexual'), the psychological (for example emotions and reasoning) and cultural and socio-economic influences such as dressing up and flirting and so on (Doll, 2012). It is often understood narrowly as genitocentric, itself tied to the heteronormative relationship between genital sex and reproduction. Yet it encapsulates a range of practices that bring sensual pleasure and fulfil wants and desires, such as the agglomeration of practices that are subsumed under the umbrella term BDSM (indicatively Weiss, 2011; Ortmann and Sprott, 2013). 'Intimacy' refers to involvement in close and interpersonal relations. It can be a feature of diverse relationships, from those that are sexual, or with strong close personal friendship bonds, or characterised by physical and emotional closeness, to those where a particular relation or facet of life is shared closely, such as close work relationships. It encompasses a spectrum of emotions, needs and activities ranging from feelings of caring, closeness and affection (that can go with long-term companionship) through to 'romance', where an individual 'idealises' a person(s) (Ehrenfeld et al, 1997). Intimacy is to a degree conceived in gendered terms: if men tend to define it more in physical terms, women usually emphasise more its emotional content (O'Brien et al, 2012). It is often conceived as two people sharing intimacy rather than a larger number and is constituted subjectively as a value that is owned or shared with others, although equally it is sometimes seen as an arena that reinforces oppressive conventions of private–public divides and 'compulsory monogamy' (Bersani and Phillips, 2008; Heckert, 2010; Musial, 2013).

These three conceptualisations – age/older, sex/sexuality and intimacies – intersect in complex ways. For example, the prevailing assumption that sexual relationships involve shared intimacy fails to recognise 'fuck buddies' or so-called casual relationships for mutual sexual gratification – though intimacy is sometimes used to describe a particular event without relationship – 'they were intimate' (Wentland and Reissing, 2014). Likewise, sex and age often enmesh in complex ways, though these linkages too often involve mutually reinforcing negative representations. Decline in sexual capacity – often reduced to coital/genital function – is associated with ageing and later life as a standard correlation as opposed to a graduated contingency. Drawing in other intersections, the relationship between sexual capacity and potency is a significant feature of masculinity and therefore sexual capacity is considered more challenging for men, given fears of loss of status and greater reluctance than women to seek help concerning sexual and relationship problems (O'Brien et al, 2012). This reflects gendered assumptions that male sexuality is more active and women's more passive that is rooted in classical sexology (indicatively Davidson and Layder, 1994; Bland and Doan, 1998). Nevertheless, the sexuality of older women could be constrained by biological changes, understood through cultural pathology as decline and loss of attractiveness. As female sexuality tends to be more associated with youth-coded beauty, older women become excluded from the sexual imaginary (Doll, 2012). In addition, women face the moral constraints of being a good wife/mother/grandmother, where being non-sexual is seen as a virtue and not a deficiency, whereby older women face moral censure for transgressing an approved ageing femininity when not acting their age (Lai and Hynie, 2011). As such, the narrative of decline is perpetuated. Since the 1970s, however, women now over 50 will have encountered the countervailing influences of feminism and challenge such culturally constituted assumptions (Bassnett, 2012; Westwood, 2016).

Even where the idea of older sexual agents meets with approval because of its contribution to well-being and self-esteem, their sexuality has been subject to a medicalised, book-keeping approach that disregards emotions and pleasures and focuses on who is still 'doing it' (Gott, 2004), in the context of declining physical capacity for genitocentric penetrative sex (see Trudel et al, 2000, as an example). However, more encouragingly, we perceive the beginnings of challenge to these negative discourses in European, Australian and US contexts and writing, which attempt to recuperate older people, including the oldest citizens (commonly care home residents) and across the spectrum of genders and sexualities, as legitimate sexual/intimate citizens (see Gott, 2004; Hafford-Letchfield, 2008; Bauer et al, 2012; Doll, 2012; Simpson et al, 2016, 2017; Villar et al, 2014). The purpose of elaborating these brief examples is to underline that a focus on sex and intimacy in later life involves the recognition of intersections both within and beyond the conceptual constituents of the series focus. Lives are not lived in sexual, intimate or aged based singularities, but in complex differentiated yet overlapping and intertwined experiences with myriad intersections, such as class, race/ethnicity, gender, disability, embodiment and affect (Simpson, 2015).

It is this rich patina of experience and knowledge creation that this series seeks to elucidate, working outward from a critical focus on the core concerns of sex/sexuality, intimacy and ageing, and providing the space for innovative and high-quality scholarship that can inform institutions, policy, professional practice, current and future research and older people experiencing this focus as lived experience and not simply subject of inquiry. The vision behind the series is summarised in the following eight points:

- It will put the sex back into sexuality (and into ageing). This arises from the observation that while sexuality studies has progressed considerably over the last 40 years (Fischer and Seidman, 2016), its development as an intellectual field of enquiry has to some extent dampened the subversive character of a focus on the 'messy physicality' of sexual pleasure. Put simply, there is lots of scholarship about sexuality, but less focus on the pleasures of sex. There is an aspiration that this series might be one avenue by which that can in a small way be corrected. Putting the 'sex' back into 'sexuality' is part of an agenda to recuperate older people to continue to be recognised as sexual citizens (or more specifically to have the choice to be sexual agents or not). As such, this series can support the vanguard of an intellectual project that will establish sex in later life as a serious yet neglected political issue and thus stimulate and advance debate. If what is at stake in understanding current experience is the impediments and constraints to choice and pleasure, embodied sensual practice and agency must constitute part of the site of scholarship.

- It will promote and offer an avenue for critically engaged work on the subject matter, whether it is empirical and theoretical-philosophical, from across the social sciences, humanities and cultural studies, incorporating scientific and aesthetic insights. An essential part of the project is that assumptions, claims and received knowledge about sex and intimacy in later life are always questioned, challenged and subject to critical review. This is the means by which both extant knowledge is tested, refined and strengthened or rejected, and new knowledge is produced. A critical frame also offers the opportunity to move beyond traditional academic frames – insofar as a book series allows – in presenting new ideas, evidence and conjectures.
- It will emphasise the value of multidisciplinary and interdisciplinary approaches to sex and intimacy in late life. Though the series is open to critical research studies from specific disciplinary positions, such as sociology, psychology or gerontology, it recognises the value of multidisciplinary studies that draw on more than one discipline or field, and interdisciplinary studies that cut across and suture together different disciplines, perspectives and approaches in understanding the complexity of older people and their sexual and intimate lives. This extends to recognising the value of the interweaving of social science, aesthetic and critical approaches across paradigm and disciplinary boundaries.
- It will recognise the value of different approaches that foreground the experiential and/or empirical and/or theoretical landscapes of sex and intimacy in later life, whether they form layered responses to a question or are presented as discrete levels of analysis.
- It will have an international focus, recognising global differences, inequalities; there is value in both the specificity and depth afforded regional, national and locally based studies but there should be acknowledgement of supranational, international and global contexts to phenomena, trends and developments and political, cultural and social responses. It should be acknowledged that the emergent knowledge on

sex, intimacy and later life has been generated mostly within academies of the Global North, but it does not follow that this necessarily implies progress in comparison to other parts of the globe. It also recognises that there are inherent difficulties of resourcing, organisation and common conceptualisation in the development of international projects with a global reach, and these difficulties are unevenly distributed across the globe. In some parts of the globe, researching this focus is not simply difficult but inherently risky to those who might be researched or researched with intolerance, hostility and lack of recognition. Genuine attempts at a global research agenda require properly distributed and balanced strategies for collaboration to meet relevant constraints and challenges. There should be both attention to the seeds of emergent scholarship in the Global South, and sensitivity to the tendency of Western scholarship to reflect a bias towards a 'colonial' approach to knowledge production. Notwithstanding the tendency for scholarship to focus on the Global North and particularly North America, Europe and Australasia, the series seeks – in a small way – to promote international understandings. This is achieved through the conviction that cross-cultural and spatial perspectives, drawing from insight and evidence across the globe, can contribute to better understandings of experience and avenues for research, policy and practice and reflection.
- It will allow for language, labels and categories that emerge from partial geographical and cultural contexts in the development of scholarship to be questioned, adapted, resisted and brought into relief with alternatives and oppositions in how age, sex, sexuality and intimacy are conceived.
- It will recognise and explore the constraints on and complications involved in expression of sexual/intimate citizenship as an older person and across a spectrum of sexual and gender identities, interrogating and challenging stereotypes of older people as prudish or sex-negative and post-sexual. Equally, the series seeks to explore, examine and advocate sex-positive approaches to sex and intimacy in later life that can help empower, enable and support older people's sexual and intimate relations.
- Finally, it will be accessible to readers in order to inform public understanding, academic study, intellectual debate, professional practice and policy development. This is an ambitious agenda to set for any enterprise, and the series hopes only to make modest contributions to it. Nevertheless, the series has been born of a conviction that unless this sort of agenda is adopted, the experience everyone shares of growing old will always be unnecessarily impoverishing and incapacitating. At the core of this series, and what it should exemplify, is the flourishing that arises from older sexual agents making choices, giving and enjoying pleasure and recognising options and experiences that are open to them as they age.

Note

1 The long full version of what has been called the 'alphabet soup' of sexual identities LGBTIQAPGNGFNBA ('Lesbian', 'Gay', 'Bisexual', 'Trans', 'Intersex', 'Questioning', 'Curious', 'Asexual', 'Pansexual', 'Gender Non-conforming', 'Gender-Fluid', 'Non-Binary' and 'Androgynous'). This list is neither exhaustive nor does it take on non-Western sexual identities and cultures that should not be assumed to be equivalent in their conception.

References

Age UK (2019) As STIs in older people continue to rise, Age UK calls to end the stigma about sex and intimacy in later life [online], Available from: https://www.ageuk. org.uk/latest-press/articles/2019/october/as-stis-in-older-people-continue- to-rise-ageuk-calls-to-end-the-stigma-about-sex-and-intimacy-in-later-life/.

Bassnett, S. (2012) *Feminist Experiences: The Women's Movement in Four Cultures*, Routledge.

Bauer, M., Fetherstonhaugh, D., Tarzia, L., Nay, R., Wellman, D. and Beattie, E. (2012) 'I always look under the bed for a man': needs and barriers to the expression of sexuality in residential aged care – the views of residents with and without dementia, *Psychology and Sexuality*, 4(3): 296–309.

Bersani, L. and Phillips, A. (2008) *Intimacies*, Chicago University Press.

Bland, L. and Doan, L. (1998) *Sexology in Culture: Labelling Bodies and Desires*, Polity Press.

Bodley-Tickell, A.T., Olowokure, B., Bhaduri, S., White, D.J., Ward, D., Ross, J.D.C., Smith, G., Duggal, H.V. and Gould, P. (2008) Trends in sexually transmitted infections (other than HIV) in older people: analysis of data from an enhanced surveillance system, *Sexually Transmitted Infections*, 84: 312–17.

Chao, J.-K., Lin, Y.-C., Ma, M.-C., Lai, C.-J., Ku, Y.-C., Kuo, W.-H. and Chao, I.-C. (2011) Relationship among sexual desire: sexual satisfaction and quality of life in middle-aged and older adults, *Journal of Sex and Marital Therapy*, 37(5): 386–403.

Cronin, A. and King, A. (2010) Power, inequality and identification: exploring diversity and intersectionality amongst older LGB adults, *Sociology*, 44(5): 876–92.

Davidson, J.O. and Layder, D. (1994) *Methods, Sex, Madness*, Routledge.

Doll, G.A. (2012) *Sexuality and Long-term Care: Understanding and Supporting the Needs of Older Adults*, Health Professions Press.

Drench, M.E. and Losee, R.H. (1996) Sexuality and the sexual capabilities of elderly people, *Rehabilitation Nursing*, 21(3): 118–23.

Ehrenfeld, M., Tabak, N., Bronner, G. and Bergman, R. (1997) Ethical dilemmas concerning the sexuality of elderly patients suffering from dementia, *International Journal of Nursing Practice*, 3(4): 255–9.

Fischer, N.L. and Seidman, S. (eds) (2016) *Introducing the New Sexuality Studies* (3rd edn), Routledge.

Foucault, M. (1977) *Discipline and Punish: The Birth of the Prison*, Penguin.

Foucault, M. (1978) *The History of Sexuality, Volume 1: An Introduction*, Penguin.

Gott, M. (2004) *Sexuality, Sexual Health and Ageing*, McGraw-Hill Education.

Hafford-Letchfield, P. (2008) 'What's love got to do with it?': developing supportive practices for the expression of sexuality, sexual identity and the intimacy needs of older people, *Journal of Care Services Management*, 2(4): 389–405.

Hancock, A.-M. (2016) *Intersectionality: An Intellectual History*, Oxford University Press.

Heckert, J. (2010) *Love without Borders? Intimacy, Identity and the State of Compulsory Monogamy* [online], Available from: http://theanarchistlibrary.org/libr ary/jamieheckert-love-without-borders-intimacy-identity-and-the-state- of-compulsory-monogamy.

Hill Collins, P. and Bilge, S. (2016) *Intersectionality*, Polity Press.

Lai, Y. and Hynie, M. (2011) A tale of two standards: an examination of young adults' endorsement of gendered and ageist sexual double standards, *Sex Roles*, 64(5–6): 360–71.

Lindau, S.T., Schumm, P., Laumann, E.O., Levinson, W., O'Muircheartaigh, C.A. and Waite, L.J. (2007) A study of sexuality and health among older adults in the United States, *New England Journal of Medicine*, 357: 762–74.

Musial, M. (2013) Richard Sennett and Eva Illouz on the tyranny of intimacy: intimacy tyrannised and intimacy as a tyrant, *Lingua Ac Communitas*, 23: 119–33.

O'Brien, K., Roe, B., Low, C., Deyn, L. and Rogers, S. (2012) An exploration of the perceived changes in intimacy of patients' relationships following head and neck cancer, *Journal of Clinical Nursing*, 21(17–18): 2499–508.

Ortmann, D. and Sprott, R. (2013) *Sexual Outsiders: Understanding BDSM Sexualities and Communities*, Rowman and Littlefield.

Rahman, M. and Jackson, S. (2010) *Gender and Sexuality: Sociological Approaches*, Polity Press.

Rich, A. (1981) *Compulsory Heterosexuality and Lesbian Experience*, Onlywomen Press.

Simpson, P. (2015) *Middle-aged Gay Men, Ageing and Ageism: Over the Rainbow?* Palgrave Macmillan.

Simpson, P., Almack, K. and Walthery, P. (2018a) 'We treat them all the same': the attitudes, knowledge and practices of staff concerning old/er lesbian, gay, bisexual and trans residents in care homes, *Ageing & Society*, 38(5): 869–99.

Simpson, P., Brown Wilson, C., Brown, L., Dickinson, T. and Horne, M. (2016) The challenges of and opportunities involved in researching intimacy and sexuality in care homes accommodating older people: a feasibility study, *Journal of Advanced Nursing*, 73(1): 127–37.

Simpson, P., Horne, M., Brown, L.J.E., Dickinson, T. and Torkington, K. (2017) Older care home residents, intimacy and sexuality, *Ageing and Society*, 37(2): 243–65.

Simpson, P., Wilson, C.B., Brown, L.J., Dickinson, T. and Horne, M. (2018b) 'We've had our sex life way back': older care home residents, sexuality and intimacy, *Ageing & Society*, 38(7): 1478–501.

Stenner, P., McFarquhar, T. and Bowling, A. (2011) Older people and 'active ageing': subjective aspects of ageing actively, *Journal of Health Psychology*, 16(3): 467–77.

Trudel, G., Turgeon, L. and Piché, L. (2000) Marital and sexual aspects of old age, *Sexual and Relationship Therapy*, 15(4): 381–406.

Villar, F., Celdrán, M., Fabà, J. and Serrat, R. (2014) Barriers to sexual expression in residential aged care facilities (RACFs): comparison of staff and residents' views, *Journal of Advanced Nursing*, 70(11): 2518–27.

Weeks, J. (2010) *Sexuality* (3rd edn), Routledge.

Weiss, M. (2011) *Techniques of Pleasure: BDSM and the Circuits of Sexuality*, Duke University Press.

Wentland, J.J. and Reissing, E. (2014) Casual sexual relationships: identifying definitions for one-night stands, booty calls, fuck buddies and friends with benefits, *The Canadian Journal of Human Sexuality*, 23(3): 167–77.

Westwood, S. (2016) *Ageing, Gender and Sexuality: Equality in Later Life*, Routledge.

Ylanne, V. (ed.) (2012) *Representing Aging: Images and Identities*, Palgrave Macmillan.

Zaninotto, P., Falaschetti, E. and Sacker, A. (2009) Age trajectories of quality of life among older adults: results from the English longitudinal study of ageing, *Quality of Life Research*, 18(10): 1301–9.

Foreword

Raffaella Ferrero Camoletto, University of Turin

For a long time, later-life sexuality was often suppressed, trivialised, or condemned, with older adults portrayed – both in public and clinical arenas – as naturally experiencing declining sexual desire and functioning. In more recent decades, however, there has been a marked shift in cultural and scholarly discourse, positioning sexuality as a salient component of healthy ageing and overall lifelong well-being. This evolution has been propelled by the confluence of two noteworthy developments: the commercial release of Viagra in 1998, subsequently followed by other 'sexuopharmaceuticals', and the emergence of a widespread rhetoric advocating active and healthy ageing.

Pharmaceutical interventions – including erectile medications such as Viagra and a range of hormone treatments – become crucial lenses through which we can re-examine not only sexual function in older adults, but also the broader politics of health, age and commercial profit. Where once older adults' sexual concerns were minimised or ignored by healthcare professionals, we now see an explosion of 'therapeutic' discourses and treatments that promise indefinite vitality. 'Sexual enhancement' products have helped construct new expectations of ongoing sexual performance well into advanced ages, reversing older stereotypes of seniors as asexual or uninterested in intimacy.

While there is a welcome shift in public perceptions – ageing need not denote the end of sexual enjoyment – it is important to point to the ambivalent legacy of what might be termed the 'Viagra era'. In particular, there is a caution that a narrow, heteronormative and youth-focused paradigm is being extended: one that privileges penetrative intercourse as the hallmark of successful ageing, often at the expense of more diverse or adaptive expressions of bodily pleasure.

Within this evolving scenario, this timely and thought-provoking edited collection addresses the challenge to the notion that older adults are necessarily desexualised or 'post-sexual' subjects. Building on foundational research in social gerontology, feminist and queer theory, the editors and contributors offer a powerful intervention into the dominant narratives that surround sexuality, intimacy and the life course. What emerges is a polyvocal conversation about how ageing bodies are reimagined, how markets and medical interventions shape sexual possibilities, and how new frameworks of sexual citizenship might open up spaces for people in later life to flourish.

The introduction lays out the conceptual terrain: it questions why the 'misery narrative' of inevitable sexual decline still wields such power, even as contemporary research consistently shows that many older people continue to value, and engage in, forms of erotic or intimate practice. The term 'resocialisation' or 'resexualisation' is introduced here to capture a dual process: the disruption of stereotypes that depict ageing as a trajectory of waning desire and capacity, and the emergence of new possibilities for sexual self-definition beyond reproductive or strictly genitocentric frameworks. Rather than presuppose that sexuality in old age is homogeneous, the Introduction emphasises the diversity of erotic experiences, the intersections of gender and sexuality, and the structural inequalities – around class, race/ethnicity, and disability – that profoundly shape the experience of ageing.

Building on this nuanced perspective, the concluding reflections revisit the persistent themes that thread through the volume as a whole, proposing a broad research agenda and policy manifesto for a 'resensualisation' or 're-enchantment' of older adulthood. These reflections insist that robust future scholarship must attend to inequality – if resexualisation is to avoid becoming the preserve of those with wealth, access to healthcare, or certain forms of cultural capital, it must actively confront how race, gender, sexuality, class and disability intersect to produce disparate experiences of ageing and intimacy. Similarly, the medical domain must become more inclusive, less paternalistic, and more open to collaborative, community-based approaches that value older adults as knowledgeable agents of their own sexual health. There is also a call for more creative methodological frameworks in the study of later-life sexuality: from ethnographies of sexual subcultures in long-term care settings, to participatory action research that engages older adults in shaping the questions and solutions they deem relevant.

One of the core messages in the volume is its invitation to move beyond a purely biomedical conversation about the 'fixes' or 'declines' of the ageing sexual body. The editors underscore that a truly emancipatory vision of sexuality in later life demands rethinking assumptions about erotic capacity, desirability and success. Reflecting on how existing scholarship has often prioritised the experiences of middle-class, white, heterosexual cisgender men, they point out that critical, intersectional, and queer perspectives can enlarge our sense of what sexual flourishing might look like for multiple constituencies. Beyond mere inclusion, the goal is to foster open dialogues that question normative standards: for instance, why should penetration remain the gold standard of sexual expression? What role might digital technologies, such as dating apps or online communities, play in carving out new 'interpretive communities' of mid- and later-life sexuality? And how can healthcare professionals, social workers and policy-makers cultivate a climate where older people feel emboldened to articulate desires and preferences that exceed or disrupt conventional frameworks?

Moreover, in a landscape increasingly shaped by consumer-driven healthcare, the contributors collectively urge us to remain vigilant about how discourses of 'healthy ageing' can inadvertently marginalise those who do not fit ableist or heteronormative ideals. Pharmaceutical resexualisation is not inherently emancipatory if it merely imposes a new set of pressures on older adults – pressure to maintain youthful performance metrics, or to consume costly interventions. A more equitable approach would foreground choice, autonomy and a holistic notion of sexual well-being. Such an approach is arguably just as relevant for the younger cohorts who will enter older adulthood in the coming decades, potentially carrying with them a legacy of activism around gender and sexual diversity. By intersecting these generational trends with current transformations in global demographics, this volume paves the way for further comparative research across regions and cultural contexts.

In sum, this edited collection seeks neither to romanticise ageing nor to deny that bodily changes can prompt shifts in one's sexual life. Instead, it proposes that these shifts need not be pathologised or passively accepted. Later-life sexuality is less a biological inevitability than a sociocultural narrative, open to intervention, resistance and creative rearticulation. By weaving together sociological, anthropological and critical gerontological perspectives, this volume stands as a testament to the idea that 'resocialising' the ageing body can be an empowering project – one that resituates older individuals as active, complex protagonists of their erotic lives. Ultimately, it issues a call for ongoing interdisciplinary research, policy advocacy and innovative practice. If society is to truly embrace older people's sexual citizenship, we must continue to dismantle desexualising myths, question the partial solutions offered by pharmaceutical culture, and cultivate a richer vocabulary for pleasure, desire and intimacy in later life.

1

Introduction: Themes, issues and chapter synopses

Paul Reynolds, Paul Simpson and Trish Hafford-Letchfield

Defining resexualisation

It seems that much scholarship on later life sexuality has focused on the misery narrative of loss and lack that is desexualisation. In contrast, this edited collection turns attention to different aspects of and possibilities for sexual and intimate citizenship, which can involve agency in a narrative of resexualisation of people in later life and beyond the cisgender heteronormative benchmark. The concept of resexualisation is closely tied to that of 'sexual citizenship', which, reflecting its multiform character, appears in various guises throughout this volume. Sexual citizenship (or who counts as one) has probably existed since antiquity, though is historically and culturally variable (Foucault, 1976) and has been theorised in more recent times in various ways. Weeks (1998) has defined it as representing the juncture between private claims to space and autonomy and public claims to sexual/bodily rights, especially in relation to newer socio-sexual subjectivities and body politics that claim value for sexual difference and diversity in erotic and intimate life. Also stressing the possibilities for agency, Plummer has defined sexual citizenship as: 'control over and respect for our bodies, feelings, representations, identities, relationships and erotics' (Plummer, 2003: 39). Striking a critical note, Evans (1993) and Bell and Binnie (2002) have noted its inequalities and exclusions (around intersecting issues of class, race, gender, sexuality), and arising from capitalist structures and discourse, concerning who can claim a legitimate version of it. More recently, Richardson (2017) has attempted to de-centre the Western-centric character of sexual citizenship and rights by looking at critiques of the atomistic, choosing individual available from within global South and other geo-political contexts. For a glimpse into forms of sexual citizenship in the global South and East that are critical of and dialogic with Western and global North hegemony, see the volume in this book series by Ghisyawan et al (2024).

We can see glimpses of most of the definitions just mentioned – assertion of various rights and the value of sexual differences, and the material and cultural inequalities in such a project – etched throughout this volume. Indeed, this is reflected in the chapters on non-monogamy and kink that reflect new, even queerer social experiments in living, and reversals of hegemonic discourse to claim legitimate sexual status in 'real' life and 'reel life' (filmic and other cultural representations), as well as in the online world. We can also see how signs of a new aesthetics concerning various social groups can help resexualise diverse older people and thus undergird their claims to sexual citizenship, as well as remarkable resexualising practices concerning sex work as care. As intimated, asserting and deploying such claims to recognition, respect and rights are far from equally available.

The aforementioned focus on resexualisation (and the allied concepts of sexual citizenship and rights) raises two difficulties: the problem of understanding the knowledge and research base from which such an enterprise begins, which frames what resexualisation might mean and involve; and an understanding of what 'resexualisation' of itself might signify as a concept.

One of the main difficulties of writing to such a theme is that it is a relatively nascent focus of research in both studies on sex and intimacy and on the lives of people in later life. Sex and intimacy in later life has been comparatively under-researched or assumed derivative of a standardised life course in its representation in the disciplines of social gerontology, socio-cultural, social psychological or sexuality studies up to the turn of the 21st century. The developing focus of research in the area has been prevalence and incidence studies on factors constraining older people's sex lives – auditing the current, impoverished state of affairs (for critical discussions, see Simpson et al, 2018; Steckenrider, 2022). Explorations of ways of enabling sex and intimacy have been restricted to limited exercises in therapeutic health and well-being including the 'how-to' or 'self-help' market (indicatively, Grant, 2018; McCarthy and McCarthy, 2022). These contributions often rest uncritically on a life stage or life cycle model of ageing that presumes a youthful peak and then slow decline from sexual or sensual relations as people age (this is covered in detail in Simpson et al, 2021). These foundations neither address the diversity of the experience of later life nor the structural and cultural conditions of desexualisation that produce rather than simply reflect life course change. Hence Volumes 1 (*Sex and Diversity in Later Life*, Hafford-Letchfield et al, 2021) and 2 (*Desexualisation in Later Life*, Simpson et al, 2021) of the 'Sex and Intimacy in Later Life' series, of which this is a companion volume.

The failure to recognise diversity has several palpable weaknesses. It assumes a marked 'life stage' model of later life that is based on the naturalised developmental model that derives from the characteristics of the development of modern capitalist industrial societies, and is conditioned by their notions of health, lifestyles and choices and structural forms and features in such areas as work/employment and family. (Indicative for discussions of the life course, see: Elder et al, 2003; Elder and Giele, 2009; Mayer, 2009; Heikkinen, 2011 and Ferraro and Schafer, 2017.) Often there is insufficient recognition of the very different global contexts to life course, as well as diversifying change in structural forms, such as family and work or consideration of how political changes such as the post-war shift from welfarism to neo-liberalism and deindustrialisation impacts upon life course experience. Also, that experience can be different depending on intersecting variables such as race and ethnicity, class or income/wealth distribution, gender and disability, and importantly, different sexualities beyond heteronormative sexual representations of sexual identity, relations, behaviours and practices and their genitocentric assumptions about what sex involves. These contextual features challenge life stage models of ageing, just as medical developments and health technologies challenge how people experience later life. The 'picture' is more complex than a staged model can reflect.

The prevailing stereotypical presumptions about moving into later life involve several questionable claims: that sexual desires and appetites reduce in intensity with age; that genitocentric sexual function and possible compromises with age directly relate to diminished sexual capacity and appetite; that ageing bodies and minds reduce in sexual attractiveness; that a genitocentric model of sex and sexuality is a common central focus and that these factors follow a medically authoritative model of 'natural' ageing (see Simpson et al, 2021 for an elaborated discussion). Rather than take these features as a given, 'natural' characterisation of ageing into later life, we have conceived them as cultural and political in their development and imposition as orthodoxy, in the construction of 'knowledge' and concerning sex and sexual involvement. Hence the use of the term 'desexualisation' as a quite specific exercise of professional knowledges and discursive regimes, instantiated in institutional settings and by those producing health, education, care and welfare to those experiencing later life, and populating public consciousness with their authoritative voices. Here, Michel Foucault's analyses of 'mad, bad, and sad' constitutions of mental health, criminality and health expose the mechanics by which pathology and prejudice capture public understandings above enquiring science and deliberative debate (Foucault, 1976, 1984a, 1984b, 1995, 2001a, 2001b, 2002, 2003, 2009, 2018).

In Volume 2 (Simpson et al, 2021: 1–2), we described desexualisation by noting (and it is worth repeating at length):

> Older people [aged 50 and over] … remain the subject of stereotyping as non-sexual or 'post-sexual' (Simpson et al, 2018) … that appears endemic in late modern societies and marks limits to who counts, age-wise, as a legitimate sexual being (Gatling et al, 2017).

> [Ageist erotophobia] … invokes widespread subconscious fear and/or denial of older people as sexual beings … there is a tendency to fall back on naturalised developmentalist fallacies (Moore and Reynolds, 2018) that represent ageing as a desexualising process, which also represent a persistent pathology. Older people's sexuality and sexual lives, … are still generally regarded with disdain, ignored or else seen as requiring interventions focused on health and risk rather than pleasure and quality of life (Garrett, 2014; Gott, 2004; Hafford-Letchfield, 2008; Villar et al, 2014).
>
> Ageism, with its associated stigmas (commonly referring to wrinkles, changing body shape, loss of physical capacity and lack of interest), prejudices and pathologies, over-associate age with loss and misery (Calasanti and King, 2019) … the factors just noted work together to feed a range of devaluing reactions [that] … range from feelings of disgust at the thought or sight of frail bodies to the infantilisation of older people's sexuality and a complete conceptual disconnect between ageing and sex (Gott, 2004; Hockey and James, 1993; Simpson et al, 2018). Yet, the literature exploring ageing sexuality that seeks to distinguish the challenges to older people who wish to enjoy sex from the desexualising discursive nexus that is imposed upon them appears relatively limited (DeLamater, 2012).

As we claim, desexualisation is experienced to different degrees, materially and culturally, through structured inequalities in race/ethnicity, class, gender, sexuality, and disability. It is also experienced in the way the 'naturalised' life stage model describes the impact of ageing, such as menopause or less reliable erectile function. These 'trends' reflect a strong association of sex with (heteronormative) genitocentric, penetrative sex as the apex of sex – with penetrative orgasm the 'primary' sexual practice. The process of desexualisation retains a strong sexological and historical impetus for sex to be described in discreet, gendered roles (males penetrate, women are penetrated) and reproduction as strongly associated with sexual practice (Bland and Doan, 1998). Against this traditional weight of orthodoxy, post-1960s cultural change and the development of reliable sexual technologies have allowed sexual practice to be conceived more as a choice than determination, opening up diversity as a real possibility of experience. This 'one-size-fits-all' conception of sex carries with it a centrality of function that is predicated on assumptions of decline with age and fails to account for a wide range of variables and alternative practices that might compromise its authority. Recognition of choice and diversity offers the possibility of alternatives.

This narrative of diversity points towards desexualisation, as experienced by people in later life, as not a natural or pre-given result of the life course.

Instead, it is produced through representational restrictions or fetishised forms of sexual knowledge and cultures, which limit public discursive practices and spaces for expression that encourage understanding, critical engagement with the 'norm' and the possibilities of choice and difference. There are specific forms of 'ageist erotophobia' that encourage self-policing and the normalisation of how erotic pleasures and desires are conceived and articulated into what is practiced or expressed erotically in a diminished or conventional form (see Simpson et al, 2018). Social institutions that are focused on later life, such as care institutions, are by their very construction underpinned by assumptions of reduced sexual desire and practice (if any). So, sex and intimacy in later life becomes discursively limited and subject to a hostile aesthetic ranging from distaste to disgust (Moore and Reynolds, 2016). This persists despite that those now entering later life are the 'baby boomer' generation of the 1960s, some of whom took an active part in the cultural disruption of conservative norms in their youth and do not conform to traditional notions and moral imperatives concerning how later life should be lived.

Building on that analysis, it is helpful to have a similar approach to describe the obverse – resexualisation. However, this is where the second difficulty with this enterprise becomes evident – conceiving resexualisation and what it means. To desexualise implies that there was sex that has been diminished. That cannot be assumed, since a progressive approach to sex and intimacy in later life has to give respect to those who may be asexual, or have always had comparatively low sex drives, or whose energies are directed elsewhere. Resexualisation is an explicit rejection of desexualisation as the product of a cultural and political ensemble of structures and their processes. It should not be an imposition of an alternative, and should emphasise that any sexual agenda involves choices, with the enabling and understanding of these choices as a primary goal. This involves also a choice not to have sex and to redefine what counts as sexual.

Further, any progressive approach to sex and intimacy in later life should account for or give space to forms of intimacy that bind people together relationally but are not sexual in character, such as 'Platonic' companionship. (This point is taken up in Chapter 8.) Hence the importance of resexualisation being enabling and in the present context emancipatory, but not constituting in and of itself a new orthodoxy. Notwithstanding the need to break down the ideological and representational power of desexualising discourses, there has to be space for those who enter later life whose mature reflection is that their ageing has led to less interest in sex. While it is important to first challenge and deconstruct the powerful structures and discourses of desexualisation to enable alternatives into the public consciousness and debate, it is then, again, a matter of choice.

A further issue with the conception of resexualisation is that it is an elusive construct since it requires recognition of diversity and plurality as features of sexual and erotic thinking and understandings in later life. Given the plurality and diversity in bodies, identities, pleasures and desires, relations, practices and socio-cultural contexts and conjunctures, any notion of resexualisation is first constituted in abstract criteria. Indicatively, this encompasses choice, sensual practices, and their environments, relational and orientational preferences and ethical notions of legitimacy and il/legitimacy in what should or not be practiced. These criteria then provide a conceptual schema to apply to and evaluate concrete instantiations within people's later lives within their particular circumstances and contexts. These might range from reconceived living and relationship arrangements such as group living and polyamorous relationships to therapeutic services such as sexological counselling or sexual surrogacy. Resexualisation will invariably mean different starting points, approaches and aims in different cultures that have different forms and customs for sex and intimacy. This might best be conceived in Raymond Williams's (2005) conception of the dominant culture being supplemented and challenged by both residual cultures from the past and emergent cultures for the future. This way of thinking shows that cultural dominance – hegemonic in character – is not of itself continuous, self-reproducing and omnipotent. Beneath dominant ideas and their prevalence in public and media discourse, different ideas and practices might be being practiced and enjoyed or experimented with, that do not always visibly challenge dominant representations and ideas but do reject or displace them at the level of private lives. Here, Williams's description of hegemony is useful in characterising the terms of cultural ebb and flow – and the possibilities of challenging orthodoxy:

> A lived in hegemony is always a process. It is not, except analytically, a system or a structure. It is a realised complex of experiences, relationships, and activities, with specific and changing pressures and limits. In practice, that is, hegemony can never be singular. Its internal structures are highly complex, as can readily be seen in any concrete analysis. Moreover (and this is crucial, reminding us of the necessary thrust of the concept), it does not just passively exist as a form of dominance. It has continually to be renewed, recreated, defended and modified. It is also continually resisted, limited, altered, challenged by pressures not at all its own. (Williams, 1977: 112–13)

The balances of strategies and tactics employed to disrupt dominant cultures will be distinctive to each cultural context, whether through public/political lobbying for legal change and changes to public policy and provision, or the emergence of alternative 'ruptures' to dominant cultures. Think of 'soft kink' and 'Fifty Shades of Grey', which can both raise alternative agendas but be incorporated into existing narratives and forms.) Alternatively, they can be political responses to the sectoral interests of social institutions such as religions, specific interest groups with strong convictions as to social norms and traditions, corporate and commercial entities whose commodification of sex, as represented in norms, is a central interest, or the institutional and professional organisation of care, health and welfare.

At the same time, and recognising the power of global late modernity and its impositions on global diversity in cultures and societies, there will be a common architecture of recognising and seeking change in extant hostile or indifferent concrete circumstances and contexts. One common starting point is evident here and in much critical work on sexuality, with the analysis of desexualisation not as natural, normal, or a bio-medical, life stage and developmental phenomena, but as a limiting socio-cultural construction tied to dominant orthodoxies and the interests who propagate and benefit from them. Whether evolved though the interests and ideologies of specific agents or a developing patina of open-ended discourses from social institutions and communities, sex and erotic intimacies have been dislocated from other activities enjoyed by people as they enter later life. There is nothing pre-figured, essential, or necessary about desexualisation. Theoretical disagreements, between Marxists, feminists, anti-racists, queer and 'crip' (theorists of disability) and other ideological positions, come from how those agents and discursive constitutions are differently characterised (indicatively, see the voluminous literature such as McRuer and Bérubé, 2006; McRuer, 2012; Drucker, 2017; Vidal-Ortiz et al, 2018; Ghodsee, 2019; Angel, 2022; Hill Collins, 2022 and Penny, 2022).

Desexualisation is a socio-cultural process, and as all such processes, is inculcated within individuals and groups who to varying degrees reproduce, conform, adapt to or resist. It is a political as well as a personal agenda – seeking to both change individual life-opportunities and experiences, and change social environments, institutions, cultures, processes that produce the conditions of desexualisation for self and others. In this respect, it is very much in tune with feminist critiques of the separation of personal and political within capitalist, racialist, ableist heteronormative patriarchy (indicatively, see Barnes, 2019; Davis, 2019; Hill Collins and Bilge, 2020). Personal sexual liberty is a limited proposition without wider change in the regulatory regimes and social resources that compose the structural conditions that frame sexual lives.

If resexualisation is fundamentally a matter of enabling, choice and consent are central characteristics. Choices as to individual sexual trajectories are tempered by a recognition of the imperative to ensure the space for choice for others. Constraints to others – the boundaries of sexual cultures – become a democratic and ethical prerogative for change, where restrictions should be based on valid argumentation rather than prejudice, the impositions of sectional values or the imperatives and ideologies of particular interests.

Autonomy is not just a matter of enabled and resourced choices of different sexual opportunities, but as already observed, the right not to be sexual or to enjoy purely non-sexual intimacies or to enjoy sex lives that may be limited within orthodoxy. Likewise, conventional intimacies and sexual relations should not be attacked prejudicially and should be respected as choices (if they *are* choices), if they are not ethically or politically problematic (or crucially involve reinforced social inequalities that deprive choices). If knowledge of sexual choices and opportunities are made freely available and people able to access and process them through such mechanisms of lifelong sexual edification with free access to diverse sexual knowledge, what people do with them is a matter of their choice.

The primary criterion for resexualisation is enabling agency – the choice and consent of the individual. Resexualisation involves three aspects of choice – first producing the means by which legitimate choice can be made, second that the choice is free, and third that concrete circumstances allow for that choice to be actualised. First, choice cannot be meaningfully exercised in an informational vacuum. This involves engaging with sexual literacy and the development of meaningful knowledge and pedagogy around sexual practices (Moore and Reynolds, 2021; Reynolds, 2021) beyond orthodox understandings of the boundaries of sex and sexuality. Older people can experience changes in their genital performance and capacities that influence their perception of their sexual selves. That 'mainstream' sexual orthodoxy is focused on genitocentrism in itself might be deemed to be worthy of critique, since genitocentric performance and capacity is narrowly conceived and widely variable in how it is conceived. Age is, however, one variable that can change sexual senses of performance and function, and the 'mainstream' focus on genitocentric notions of sex invariably creates uncertainty, anxiety and self-conscious sense of deficiency or lack. Wider knowledge of the diverse senses in which erotic, sensual and sexual pleasure can be enjoyed opens up opportunities for sexual fulfilment outside of this very limiting orthodoxy.

Second, it would be fallacious to expect sexual agency and choice to flourish in a context where more general social and intimate relations are otherwise. Any appeal to resexualisation requires recognition of the importance of rejecting oppressive and violent, coercive behaviours inflicted upon others, pathologies and prejudices against others (such as disabled people) whose sexual agency and choice might be differently constrained or narrowed. This also involves recognition that sexual choice should only be curtailed by rational and deliberative judgements as to the legitimacy of different acts, behaviours, relations or identities. Sexual legitimacy in this context is determined by the degree of harm to self, other and community. This may well mean prohibitions on sexual association with young people around the age of consent, or with public sexual expression, but these would be debated, regulated, and in the latter, for example, safe space for public sex might be allocated. Of course, it is a given that a resexualised later life can only come with free sexualised experience across the life course.

Finally, in this section, there is the issue of environment. This might involve rethinking the community and public space to meet and engage sexually with others, or the reshaping of the way the day is organised to enable sexual relations that are not restricted to late evenings or early mornings and associated with proximity to beds. To an extent, some of these issues of free choice, space and time and recognising diversity are practiced in particular networks or friendship groups, but resexualisation would involve opening this up so everyone is both enabled to, and feels the confidence to, consider their choices, experiment and arrive at their preferences without feeling compromised. There is no doubt that this sketch of the terms of change raises difficult questions, as to the degrees of sexual openness within a society. Issues such as: sexual aesthetics in public space, architecture and environments; public nudity or spaces for public sexual contact; the legitimacy of forms of non-coercive sex work (recognising that is in itself subject to debate); social and cultural associations that enable diverse sexual practices and relations; the disposition of time and resources that enable rich erotic and intimate lives; and the forms of knowledge and media available by which sexual expression can take place.

So, resexualisation is only intelligible if we recognise it as the obverse of desexualisation as a constructed social, cultural and political process. When we move much beyond its oppositional quality, and the bare conceptual outlines of what it might be, we find ourselves surveying a range of sometimes disparate options and choices. The coherence is in the struggle against current sexual orthodoxy, it is not to impose an alternative beyond a positive constructing of people's own decisions.

Contributions to the volume: themes and chapters in order

The different chapters in this collection reflect the concerns of emerging and established scholars (in the social sciences and humanities), activists, social work practitioners and sex educators. In light of the discussion on the conceptual challenges inherent in resexualisation, the chapters are quite varied and do not constitute a cohesive set of strategies for a more sexually free and open society. Instead, they provoke thinking on what taking desexualised later life and liberating it might look like. The volume, then, recognises the special circumstances under which sexual repression and pathology are exercised on people experiencing later life, and addresses that directly in respect of how older people and those who support a greater sexual openness and diversity from which they might make choices can begin to develop agendas for change.

Surveying the nine substantive chapters, two broad themes become apparent. First, we observe a common focus on cultures of resexualisation invoking important cultural moments, comprising a novel aesthetics, sex beyond monogamy, cinematic representations of older lesbian and gay sexual beings, and resexualisation through pharmaculture. The latter chapter is strategically placed at the start of the second part of the volume, as it bridges the theme of culture and that of technologies and practices that can (though not always or equally) enable resexualisation, comprising use of digital means/culture, internet dating, sex care workers and aids and thought-out, theoretically-informed care practices supporting older disabled people's sexuality.

Cultures of resexualisation

In Chapter 2, Feliciano Villar and Ricardo Iacub consider the broader problems of possibilities in developing a positive aesthetic of eroticism for later life. The cultural representation of sex and intimacy in later life as erotic is a central feature of shifting from the present negativity to a more positive conception of sex and intimacy. In doing so, they take account of issues of gender, age and sexual identity and relations in recognising constraints to the way dominant culture represents older lives as not aesthetically erotic. Ranging across different sexual and gender identities and cultural forms, such as pornography, they explore the constraints on positive erotic aesthetics for later life in the nexus of power and pathological discourse that imprints upon cultural representations. Simultaneously, they bring into view the possibilities for the development of an aesthetic that represents older people as erotic subjects not just for other older people but across age divisions.

In Chapter 3, Eir-Anne Edgar focuses attention on non-monogamy and older people, drawing from an array of sociological and sexual studies to analyse representations of individuals in several different films. Like Simpson and Todd in Chapter 4, she sees the possibilities that the film formats represent older people engaging in diverse sexual practices with positive portrayals that help to break down outdated and narrow stereotypes that tend to persist in mainstream film. Noting the generational changes to the composition of older people that includes 'baby boomers' of the 1960s and 1970s, she sees positive portrayals of sex and intimate creativity in later life as reflecting past lived practice and so challenging current film representations as potential audience and thus providing the impetus for films to break out of the shackles of conventional orthodoxy.

Staying in the field of cinematic representational culture, In Chapter 4, Paul Simpson and Megan Todd analyse two independently-made Canadian films, *Cloudburst* and *Gerontophilia*, to explore the possibilities for normalising old lesbian-identified women (*Cloudburst*) and old gay men (*Gerontophilia*) as legitimate sexual beings. They argue that resexualisation in both films is achieved through thought and practices open to older lesbian and gay people that challenge desexualisation, subvert stereotypes of sexlessness and involve an epistemology that enables seeing of the allure and value of older lesbian and gay selves. These depictions indicate strategies for gay men especially and lesbian-identified women who can report feeling desexualised earlier in life compared to their heterosexual peers. This chapter has an important focus on lesbians and gay men, indicative of the way in which bio-medical and conventional views of later life are limited in recognising diversity in sexual identity, relations and behaviours. Heteronormative assumptions permeate the pathologising of sex for people in later life. Simpson and Todd signpost the sense in which cultural representations offer a means by which older lesbians and gay men (and perhaps further, older diverse sexual agents) have the opportunity to use cultural forms to question the pathological framing and desexualisation of later life.

In Chapter 5, Paul Reynolds explores the problems and possibilities of alternative forms of sexual cultures in exploring how kink (often related to BDSM sexuality) might enhance and resexualise later life. While there are undoubtedly gendered and sexual features of BDSM culture that conform to more general gendered and sexual orthodoxies – departing only in practices and cultural representations – Reynolds argues that kink/BDSM offers the possibility of subverting genitocentric conceptions of sex for richer and more creative means by which erotic and sensual, sexual pleasures can be enjoyed. While kink/BDSM has, to a degree, entered public culture with filmic representations such as *Fifty Shades of Grey*, the author argues that it is important not only to see the potential of this sexual sub-culture to provide meaningful and sensual erotic experiences. It is also important to see it as part of a politics that can disrupt sexual convention and so encourage older people to experiment, experience and question their conventional understandings.

Technologies and practices of resexualisation

Providing an excellent bridge between cultures and the next section on *Technologies* in Chapter 6, Barbara Marshall explores the impact of the development of pharmaceutical technologies and products, often offering sexual enhancement and so a form of resexualisation, but in conformist medical terms on sexual functionality. With a focus on the sexuopharmaceuticals in the post-Viagra era, where new concepts of sexual 'function' and 'dysfunction' have emerged as pivotal concerns for rehabilitating ageing bodies, the chapter draws from a range of source materials to argue that gendered and sexualised ageing bodies have become lucrative resources for global pharmaceutical markets. While noting how these developments may give rise to some positive sexual representations and experiences in later life, the author is critical of how the pharmaceutical re-sexing of ageing bodies is framed by biologically reductive and implicitly ageist and heterosexist cultural politics.

Also, overlapping with the theme of cultures, in Chapter 7, Liat Ayalon and Ateret Gewirtz-Meydan explore the impact of new technologies and their cultural impacts in considering the development of the digital world for sex and intimate experience in later life. Their focus is on two questions: How do older adults use the media for love and sex? How do media represent the sexuality of older adults? The first question points to the use of digital technologies for seeking intimate partnerships and of sexual satisfaction whether through watching online content or communicating online or seeking advice and information about sex and sexuality. The second question focuses on the online representations of older people, which allows for both the imposition of conventional and orthodox representations and the possibilities afforded by alternative representations and accompanying information sources. Here, the authors survey a terrain that is constantly evolving and a prime area for both future research and for possible activism to resist desexualisation.

Chapter 8, by Christine Beasley and Mary Holmes, also focuses on digital technologies in looking specifically at older people's internet dating, and explores whether heterosexual internet dating, as a relatively new technology of intimacy, offers opportunities for moving beyond the constraints of gendered heteronormativity and for advancing gender equality within the context of resexualisation. Noting both the research focus on the young rather than older people, and the reproduction of systemic prejudice against older people as producing strong impacts of age discrimination on older people, producing the implications for their engagement in dating per se, as well in relation to internet dating. Notwithstanding the persistence of gendered hetero norms, they point to how older people can creatively subvert gendered heteronormativity, where their experiences of internet dating convert to opportunities for social change.

In Chapter 9, Nathalie Huitema and Tineke Roelofs turn attention to how resexualisation might take place through practices and arrangements in institutional contexts in examining the inclusion of sex care services in Dutch nursing home care. They note a paradigm shift in how some Dutch care institutions have shifted from medical care perspectives to holistic, person-centred care, acknowledging the sexual needs of residents. This project includes training care staff, engagement with sexologists and the service of sex care workers for individual residents. Noting how this is still relatively uncommon within a nursing home setting, they provide a discussion of how sex care services developed in institutional care and what practical implications and lessons from the experiences of care staff, residents and sex care work organisations can offer about this important development in enriching the lives of older people in care contexts.

In Chapter 10, the final chapter of Part II, Susan Gillen and Paul Reynolds provide a framework and research agenda for resexualising the lives of older disabled people. Drawing on previous work (Hafford-Letchfield et al, 2021; Simpson et al, 2021), they identify the way in which in which pathological approaches to sex and intimacy in later life are compounded by assumptions of deficiency and lack for physically, intellectually and emotionally disabled people. From there, they take queer, 'crip' and radical critiques, and importantly some recent initiatives that seek to enable disabled older people to enjoy their intimate lives, to suggest that while disabilities require recognition of specific needs, support and specific adjustments, the assumption they create sexual constraints or deficiencies are a manifestation of prejudicial orthodoxy.

Resexualisation involves an understanding of the spatial, temporal, representational, cultural and political relations, materialities and discourses by which desexualisation is constructed and sustained; a counterhegemonic strategy that dissembles these factors and pathologies and prejudices, both imposed upon and internalised; and a creative space where the nexus of sex, age and disability can be reconceived to focus on pleasure, intimate expression and productive relations and discursive constructs within changed material conditions. The authors argue that these conditions offer possibilities that would enrich and enable older disabled people (and also provide the possibilities of more general enrichment) as well as reconceptualisation of what constitutes abilities/disabilities. While a framework and agenda, it is also a provocation for other researchers to do more detailed work in this under-researched area within their particular contexts.

In sum, the chapters outlined provide a range of possibilities for resexualisation and beyond cisgender-heteronormativity that counteract dominant discourses. Drawing on various theories, they portray various possibilities and actualities across diverse contexts, invoking a range of material and discursive resources, representations, modalities and practices that visualise older people as desirable and desiring. As such, this phenomenologically rich and critically-focused, cultural-political project indicates a manifesto of sorts that will be returned to in the concluding chapter.

References

Angel, K. (2022) *Tomorrow Sex Will Be Good Again: Women and Desire in the Age of Consent*, Verso.

Barnes, E. (2019) *The Minority Body: A Theory of Disability*, Oxford University Press.

Bell, D. and Binnie, J. (2002) Sexual citizenship: marriage, the market and the military, in S. Seidman and D. Richardson (eds) *Handbook of Lesbian and Gay Studies*, Sage Publications, pp 443–58.

Bland, L. and Doan, L. (1998) *Sexology in Culture: Labelling Bodies and Desires*, Polity.

Davis, A.Y. (2019) *Women, Race & Class*, Penguin.

Elder, G.H. Jr. and Giele, J.Z. (eds) (2009) *The Craft of Life Course Research*, The Guilford Press.

Elder, G.H. Jr., Johnson, M.K. and Crosnoe, R. (2003) The emergence and development of life course theory, *Handbook of the Life Course*, Springer, pp 3–19.

Evans, D. (1993/2013) *Sexual Citizenship: The Material Construction of Sexualities*, Routledge.

Drucker, P. (2017) *Warped: Gay Normality and Queer Anti-Capitalism*, Brill.

Ferraro, K.F. and Schafer, M.H. (2017) Visions of the life course: risks, resources, and vulnerability, *Research in Human Development*, 14(1): 88–93.

Foucault, M. (1976) *The History of Sexuality Volume 1: The Will to Knowledge*, Penguin.

Foucault, M. (1984a) *The History of Sexuality Volume 2: The Use of Pleasure*, Penguin.

Foucault, M. (1984b) *History of Sexuality Volume 3: The Care of the Self*, Penguin.

Foucault, M. (1995) *Discipline & Punish: The Birth of the Prison* (2nd edn), Vintage.

Foucault, M. (2001a) *Madness and Civilisation*, (2nd edn), Routledge.

Foucault, M. (2001b) *The Order of Things: An Archaeology of the Human Sciences*, Routledge.

Foucault, M. (2002) *Archaeology of Knowledge*, Routledge.

Foucault, M. (2003) *The Birth of the Clinic: An Archaeology of Medical Perception*, Routledge.

Foucault, M. (2009) *History of Madness*, Routledge.

Foucault, M. (2018) *History of Sexuality Volume 4: Confessions of the Flesh*, Penguin.

Ghisyawan, K-N., Harley, D., Shah, S. and Simpson, P. (2024) *Later Life Sex and Intimacy in The Majority World*, Policy Press.

Ghodsee, K. (2019) *Why Women Have Better Sex Under Socialism: And Other Arguments for Economic Independence*, Vintage.

Grant, J. (2018) *Sex after Seventy: It Gets Better: The Detailed Sex Guide for Mature Thinking Adults and for Seniors*, Universe.

Hafford-Letchfield. T., Simpson. P. and Reynolds, P. (eds) (2021) *Sex and Diversity in Later Life: Critical Perspectives*, Policy Press.

Heikkinen, E. (2011) A life course approach: research orientations and future challenges, *European Review of Aging and Physical Activity*, 8: 7–12.

Hill Collins, P. (2022) *Black Feminist Thought, 30th Anniversary Edition: Knowledge, Consciousness, and the Politics of Empowerment*, Routledge.

Hill Collins, P. and Bilge, S. (2020) *Intersectionality* (2nd edn), Polity.

Mayer, K.U. (2009) New directions in life course research, *Annual Review of Sociology*, 35: 413–33.

McCarthy, B., and McCarthy, E. (2022) *Couple Sexuality After 60: Intimate, Pleasurable, and Satisfying*, Routledge.

McRuer, R. (2012) *Sex and Disability*, Durham: Duke University Press.

McRuer, R. and Bérubé, M. (2006) *Crip Theory: Cultural Signs of Queerness and* Disability, NYU Press.

Moore, A. and Reynolds, P. (2016) Against the ugliness of age: towards an erotics of the aging sexual body, *Interalia*, 11: 88–105.

Moore, A. and Reynolds, P. (2021) Advocating sexual literacy, in *Critical Sexual Literacy: Forecasting Trends in Sexual Politics, Diversity and Pedagogy*, Anthem Press, 323–32.

Penny, L. (2022) *Sexual Revolution: Modern Fascism and the Feminist Fightback*, London: Bloomsbury.

Plummer, K. (2003) *Intimate Citizenship: Private Decisions and Public Dialogues*, University of Washington Press.

Reynolds, P. (2021) Consent and sexual literacy for older people, *Desexualisation in Later Life: The Limits of Sex and Intimacy*, Policy Press, pp 17–33.

Richardson, D. (2017) *Sexuality and Citizenship*, Polity.

Simpson, P., Reynolds, P. and Hafford-Letchfield, T. (2021) *Desexualisation in Later Life: The Limits of Sex and Intimacy*, Policy Press.

Simpson, P., Brown Wilson, C., Brown, L., Horne, M. and Dickinson, T. (2018) 'We've had our sex life way back': older care home residents, sexuality and intimacy, *Ageing and Society*, 38(7): 1478–501.

Steckenrider, J. (2022) Sexual activity of older adults: we're asking the wrong questions, *Innovative Aging*, 6(Supplement 1): 500.

Vidal-Ortiz, S., Robinson, B.A. and Khan, C. (2018) *Race and Sexuality*, Polity.

Weeks, J. (1998) The sexual citizen, *Theory, Culture and Society*, 15(3–4): 35–52.

Williams, R. (1977) *Marxism and Literature*, Oxford University Press.

Williams, R. (2005) Base and superstructure in Marxist cultural theory, *Culture and Materialism*, Verso, pp 31–49.

PART I

Cultures of resexualisation

2

Can wrinkles be sexy? Possibilities and constraints for an aesthetic of eroticism in later life

Feliciano Villar and Ricardo Iacub

La arruga es bella ('wrinkles are beautiful'). This motto, coined by the Spanish fashion designer Adolfo Domínguez in the 1980s, became hugely popular (it is still today associated with him and his company) and helped him to boost a long-lasting and successful career in the fashion industry. Of course, those wrinkles referred to the creases of cotton or linen fabric that, according to him, do not have to be eliminated or ironed. On the contrary, they have to be proudly exposed since they are an intrinsic part of the natural beauty of clothes.

Can this innovative approach also be applied to other wrinkles, the unavoidable signs that time carves on our bodies and faces? And, from a more challenging perspective, can such body or face wrinkles be not just 'beautiful', but even 'sexy'? That is, can older people, as well as being respected or admired, be found sexually appealing, regardless of the age of the beholder? In this chapter we will examine such ideas, describing in which way our contemporary culture is opening incipient spaces for alternative aesthetics of eroticism in later life, and contributing to their re-sexualisation.

Thus, our goal is to explore how such 'aesthetics of eroticism in later life' are being constructed, identifying different alternatives and their underlying meanings and narratives, and analysing their possibilities and constraints (Iacub, 2006; Iacub and Villar, 2021). That is, we aim to present some ways of including older age within an aesthetic of eroticism, how such inclusion is culturally performed and what the consequences may be for older people. Even when these possibilities are more frequent within specific subcultures, and alternative aesthetic expressions emerge, and while these may, in numerous instances, perpetuate prevailing perspectives, they can also be regarded as alternatives and novel possibilities.

To do so, we will explore three different spaces. Firstly, the space of heterosexual relationships and the gendered ways they offer for keeping older people as objects of younger desire. We will discuss emerging stereotypes, such as sugar daddies or DILFs in the case of men, or cougars and MILFs in the case of women. Secondly, the space of gay subculture, and particularly the stereotypes of 'bear' and 'silver bear' as an epitome of older people as erotic figures. In this case, we will present some data coming from field research including views of both younger and older gay people. Finally, we will explore pornography as an area where such alternative aesthetics of older people are particularly prolific.

However, before exploring the spaces mentioned, it is important briefly to clarify how older age has been excluded from any aesthetic of eroticism, at least in contemporary times. Such discussion will illuminate why including older people in any aesthetic alternative may be a particularly challenging task.

The challenging task of finding an aesthetic of eroticism in later life

The word 'aesthetic' derives from the Latin *aestheticus*, and this in turn from the Greek *aisthētikós*, meaning perception, or what is registered through our senses. Aesthetics is also a traditional branch of philosophy, the one analysing how a society organises and interprets senses, perceptions and emotions, resulting in particular types of knowledge regarding what is beautiful or ugly, what is good or bad taste. In turn, such knowledge justifies emotional responses and aesthetic judgments (García-Sierra, 2019).

Culture organises, in each historical period, particular ways of aesthetic appreciation. That is, when talking about aesthetics, we talk about a situated interpretation that produces historically and culturally contingent models. Such models determine certain concepts of beauty, associated with particular ways of enjoying eroticism.

Such aesthetic models, when applied to persons, include traits and features demarcating what is beautiful and desirable, and separating them from what is deemed to be ugly and disgusting. So, it is well-known that the hegemonic and traditional trends place them in a category that excludes them from eroticism, and assigns them a non-aesthetic label. Literature on attitudes towards sexuality in later life supports this negative view. Older people are denied their value as objects of desire, they are depicted as sexually unattractive, since erotic beauty has always been associated with youthful, energetic bodies (González, 2007). As subjects of desire, when older people openly show an interest in sex, this interest may be condemned as inappropriate or seen as shameful, disgusting or laughable, evoking the 'dirty old man' category (Hillman, 2012; Gewirtz-Meydan et al, 2018).

The negative value assigned to the aesthetics of eroticism in later life (Iacub, 2006), has been naturalised in very diverse cultural origins and historical periods by associating it with different conditions, such as sin, physical disease or perversion. From this point of view, sexuality and desire are restricted to younger stages of life, unattainable for older people (both as objects and as subjects of desire), which in turn has led to the desexualisation of later life.

However, the fact that the dominant aesthetics of eroticism are cultural and historically situated also opens the door for the possibility of change, or for the coexistence with alternative social and symbolic aesthetics of eroticism including, directly or indirectly, older people. The emergence of such alternative models has to do with the loosening of strict notions of 'legitimate' sexuality and their bond with reproduction, which can be dated back to the 1960s sexual revolution in Western societies. It also has to do with a trend towards the de-standardisation and individualisation of the life course (Settersen and Tauten, 2008; Widmer et al, 2009), which has allowed for a broadening and diversification of social expectations for older people. Broader and more flexible views of sexuality, far beyond the rigid framework of reproduction and coitus and including sexual spaces traditionally considered perverse, allow for questioning of the exclusion of older people from sexuality.

Such changes do not determine or automatically create alternative aesthetics of eroticism in later life, but they are necessary conditions for them to emerge. They appear as a possibility to conceive new models that organise perception and human emotions around beauty in which sensuality and eroticism can also be associated with older people. In the following sections we identify some of these models, and their implications for the re-sexualisation of later life.

Resexualising older age: views from heterosexual relationships

Western countries have undergone a shift towards sexual permissiveness, which is reflected in more positive attitudes towards sexual behaviours that have traditionally been condemned (Smith, 2011), including those taking place in later life (Syme and Cohn, 2016).

The emergence, in the last few decades, of a positive view of older people and ageing, being the popularity of concepts such as active ageing (WHO, 2002) or successful ageing (Rowe and Kahn, 2015) in both academic and lay arenas are a good example of such a trend. This new and positive way of ageing is related to the possibility, due to a belief in the personal control of our own ageing process, of maintaining a middle-aged lifestyle for as long as one may want. Such a lifestyle would include sexual interests and activities that had been generally associated with younger people, which have led to the emergence of what some authors have labelled a 'sexy-senior' or 'sexy-oldie' discourse. This discourse depicts older people who can (and implicitly, should) keep an active (and consequently, satisfactory) sexual life until the very end of their lives (Vares, 2009; Hinchliff and Gott, 2017), resorting to medical or pharmaceutical help if difficulties are found (Marshall, 2010).

Such active sexual life is supposed to guarantee well-being and enjoyment (Smith et al, 2019).

However, it is one thing to say that older people can extend their sexual life, and attract and be attracted by other older people, but quite another thing to create new aesthetic erotic models of older people, which allow them to be the object of desire by people of any age, including younger people. This is a far more challenging task that requires deeper cultural changes, and it is the focus of this chapter.

As we will see, that creation of alternative aesthetics of eroticism in later life navigates between the traditional views of decline and asexuality and the new models of active and 'youthful', also in sexual terms, older people. At the same time, it is a deeply gendered endeavour, since the possibilities and constraints are not the same for women as for men.

Resexualising older men

Heterosexual couple relationships in which men are older than women are not strange at all. In fact, in virtually every country in the world, age gaps in heterosexual marriages show a consistent tendency for male spouses to be slightly older than their female counterparts (Gustafson and Fransson, 2015; Giuliani, 2020). Similarly, research into relationship preferences has found that irrespective of culture, men prefer younger women, with the desired age gap increasing progressively with the man's age, while women are more open to being attracted by older men (Antfolk et al, 2015). In online relationships, Bergström and Kramer (2015) found that there is a larger variation among women's preferences when compared with men's preferences, who tend to prefer younger female partners. This situation places men in a more favourable position regarding aesthetic models of eroticism in later life.

Nevertheless, we should consider that such age gaps generally do not exceed a few years. If a couple's age difference is perceived as too large (for example, an older man with a woman in her twenties or thirties), doubts about the legitimacy and romantic nature of the relationship may arise. Such doubts generally come from different sources (Villar et al, 2019). For instance, the older man can be viewed as an abusing or manipulating figure who has deceived an innocent and more immature woman, who can be considered to be seeking a paternal figure. In other cases, doubts can be mixed with a class ingredient: that is, the older man is thought to be using his financial position or social status as a way to 'buy' sex, while the younger woman is using her attractive body and sex appeal to achieve financial gains or security (Berardo et al, 1993; Gobind and du Plessis, 2015). Popular labels such as 'chickenhawk' (in gay culture), 'sugar daddy' or 'cradle snatcher' express that 'vampirising' relationship in which the older man is considered to be involved in a morally flawed relationship, in a disguised form of prostitution.

Despite such derogatory stereotypes, it is undeniable that in many couples in which the man is far older than the woman, she is truly sexually attracted by him, which suggests that there is a model or some kind of erotic beauty in older men. Unlike women, older men, especially those who are productive and wealthy, may be an object of desire well into later life (Clarke, 2018; Silva, 2019). For instance, the age-dissimilar couples interviewed by McKenzie (2015) underpinned their relationship in romantic love, a love that in some cases is even particularly 'pure' and 'blind', since it goes beyond age boundaries. However, most participants, including younger women, also underline the importance of having a physical attraction for their partner as a key ingredient in their relationship, despite the co-existence of non-bodily characteristics, such as experience, maturity or wisdom. Such sexual appeal of older men also commonly appears in studies researching 'sugar-daddy relationships'. Some younger women involved in this type of relationship, in which there is an interchange of money or gifts for sex, mentioned experience (including sexual experience), and attraction by older men as a key motive to initiate the relationship or in selecting a particular partner (Daly, 2017).

The discourse of successful ageing and maintaining an active lifestyle and healthy look, combined with some age markers that in the case of men could mean experience and maturity rather than deterioration (white hair, and wrinkles to a point) undoubtedly has helped to retain the aesthetic value of later life in men. The 'Viagra revolution' (Ferrero Camoletto, 2019), which put at bay the perils of erectile dysfunction once associated with normal ageing, has also helped to reap security and identity gains and to re-sexualise older masculine bodies. Such sexualisation remains to be associated with penetrative sex, which still keeps a hegemonic and almost 'fetish' value, and becomes a signal of good health and of successful ageing (Marshall, 2010; Sandberg, 2016).

More recently, the redefinition of masculinity in a more open, caring and emotionally-oriented way has also contributed to the emergence of new aesthetics of eroticism associated with mature men. For instance, Smith (2018) identifies a new model of masculinity called DILF ('daddy I'd like to fuck') made of combining 'bulging biceps and tender kisses'. This model adds to the traditionally masculine qualities of vigorous body, physical strength and dominance, other qualities that may even increase their attractiveness, such as sweetness, playfulness and care. In such 'domesticated masculinity', the fatherhood role is central, a role that instead of decreasing their sexual appeal, reinforces it. Thus, DILFs are affectionate parents eager to provide as much 'childcare' (or care for the younger partner) as they can (Oswald et al, 2020).

Despite that DILFs are generally middle-aged men, the presence of new sexualised masculinities more focused on 'soft qualities' potentially immune to the passing years, such as care and affection, may pave the way to the appearance of alternative masculine aesthetics of eroticism also in later life.

Resexualising older women

If, as we have seen in the previous section, culture provides some aesthetic models and examples of 'sexy older men' (models that are disseminated and reproduced by the media), the provision of similar models for women is more difficult and less frequent. In our culture, being able to preserve a youthful appearance and fit inside a definition of what is supposed to be 'attractive' is far more important for women than for men, a situation that exemplifies what Susan Sontag labelled 'the double standard of aging' (Sontag, 1997).

In light of the point just made, women seem to pay a particularly heavy price in terms of social status, visibility and sexual appeal when they age, since these qualities have been more anchored to keeping a youthful beauty than in the case of men. Accordingly, aging is associated with declining sex appeal and dating potential in women more than in men (Clarke, 2018).

Accordingly, it is perhaps unsurprising that still today, couples with large age differences in which women are older than men are perceived as far more shocking than the opposite. As an example, we may remember the case of Brigitte Macron, wife of the President of France, Emmanuel Macron (elected in 2017) and 23 years older than him. The media interest and scrutiny of this couple was far more intense than in the similar case of Ivanna Trump and Donald Trump (President of the US from 2017 to 2020 and re-elected in 2023), whose age difference was also 23 years, but in this case she was younger than him (Giuliani, 2020).

This stigmatising potential of romantic or sexual relationships in which women are older has also been found in empirical research (Collisson and Ponce de León, 2020; Vanderheiden, 2025). For instance, a common fear is that the woman could be confused with the man's mother. For men, the major problem is not having shared generational references, or the distance from peers, and remarkably, ageing and lack of beauty is mentioned far more frequently by women than by men. Younger men involved in romantic relationships with older women underline depth, life experience, maturity and security as qualities they found in their older partners.

Closely related to these types of age-discrepant relationships, in recent years we have also witnessed the appearance of new aesthetics of eroticism for older women. Some of these have appeared under the labels of 'cougar' and 'MILF'. In a sense, we will see how such 'new' aesthetics are perhaps no different from what we have already seen, and in which sense they are constrained, or even reproduce, traditional youthful aesthetics models.

The term 'cougar' has been applied to a stereotypical older woman, typically in her forties or fifties, who seeks a relationship with a younger man. Cougars have been represented in popular culture as self-confident and sexually assertive women, capable of breaking the traditional sexual script that assigned women a passive role in couple relationships (Collard, 2012; Kaklamanidou, 2012).

Some women to whom the term is attributed actually reject it because of its predatory overtones and portraying older women as animalistic and 'devouring' young male victims for their own sexual interest (Montemurro and Siefken, 2014). Such an image does not reflect the reality of age-discrepant couples, in which younger men seek relationships as actively as older women (Alarie, 2019, 2020).

Despite those negative implications, the emergence of the cougar stereotype could also suggest a new, disrupting aesthetic of mature women's eroticism. This involves open, empowered expression of sexual rights, desires and bodily autonomy as an active agent within a relationship (Vanderheiden, 2025, and, simultaneously, being younger men's object of desire and sexual fantasies (Alarie, 2020). In this context, age leaves its mark on women's bodies but does not diminish significantly their capacity for sexual attraction. On the contrary, some cougars say that being sexually assertive is a capacity they have developed with age and experience (Alarie, 2020).

Closely related to the cougar stereotype is the figure of the MILF ('mother I'd like to fuck') or 'hot mom'. This stereotype underlines, even more than in the case of cougars, the sexually desirable beauty of mature mothers. It focuses on physical appearance, rather than on identity or personality characteristics. They contradict traditional expectations attached to mothers, who were expected to keep their sexuality private, to not dress 'provocatively', and to be good role models for their children (Montemurro and Siefken, 2012). However, unlike DILFs already discussed, in whom the fact of being fathers and actively caring for their children is an important ingredient of their sexual appeal, for MILFs, being sexually desirable and being a mother are not so closely related, both aspects do not mix and boost each other (Friedman, 2014). That is, while in DILFs their fatherhood status is highly erotic, MILFs are erotic despite their motherhood status (Oswald et al, 2020).

Cougars and MILFs are a welcomed addition to create new aesthetic erotic models of later life. However, we should bear in mind that such models also have some constraints. Firstly, both cougars and MILFs are depicted as women between 30 and 50 years old. In other words, they are models for middle-aged women, rather than for older ones. Women in their 60s and beyond hardly can fit into such models. And secondly, it has been argued that cougars, and particularly MILFs, may reinforce the association of beauty with a young external look. That is, these women are sometimes portrayed as trying to remain young, masking any external sign of ageing or being desirable for their age. The message that MILFs convey, reinforced by the cosmetics and 'anti-ageing' industry (Clarke, 2010), is that 'reclaiming' a youthful appearance (that is, beauty) is possible and depends on individual effort. Consequently, MILFs represent an ideal of 'growing old without ageing' (Coupland, 2009), which may lead to what Van Bauwel (2021) has labelled a process of 'girlification' of mature and older women, a process which can be understood not as an alternative aesthetics of eroticism in later life, but as the opposite: the denial of that very possibility.

Resexualising older age: views from gay relationships

Although dominant images of gay beauty have evolved throughout history, the hegemonic aesthetics of eroticism for gay men seem to be closely associated with muscular, athletic, and hairless bodies (Drummond, 2010), thus privileging younger bodies. Clearly, gay men tend to prefer younger sexual counterparts even more frequently than heterosexual men and women (Kaufman and Chin Phua, 2003). Such models can be lived as oppression, and ageing gay men are found to make efforts to conform to that hegemonic younger model of eroticism, working against losing the aesthetic appeal of their ageing bodies (Slevin and Linneman, 2010) or defining themselves as exceptions and exemplars of a particularly 'good' way of ageing (Suen, 2017).

Nonetheless, among gay men, we also find alternative aesthetics that disrupt such dominant, youth-oriented models. Among them, the 'bear' gay subculture is particularly interesting (Quidley-Rodriguez and De Santis, 2019). According to the website 'The Ultimate Bear Resource' (http://ultimatebearlinks.pbworks.com/), bears are 'gay and bisexual men with stocky or heavyset builds, and often have hairy bodies and facial hair. Bears often exhibit an outwardly masculine appearance. The latter being the more important trait of a Bear'. Although there is not an explicit mention of age, bear culture is based on an aesthetic of maturity (Manley et al, 2007), and the bear community even differentiate subtypes such as 'Grizzly bears' (who are clearly older) and 'Polar bears' (who have white or grey 'fur' or body hair).

Bears seem to embrace an 'aesthetics of naturalism', which include the acceptance of maturity and the physical changes associated with ageing, which in turn allows for the inclusion of types beyond the hegemonic aesthetics of gay men: beyond the conventional images of muscles, youth and slenderness, bear culture can embrace older and fatter objects of desire. It celebrates what is masculine, big and heavy, but at the same time encouraging non-traditional male values, such as affection, intimacy, nurturance and interpersonal care (Hennan, 2005; Manley et al, 2007; Gough and Flanders, 2009). Such values promote body self-acceptance and resistance to ageism, but also emotionally closer social bonds, which sometimes lead to the presence of some forms of mentoring in which older bears take a protective role for younger members of their community, the 'baby bears'. In this intergenerational space appears the figure of the 'silver bear', described as an important part of the bear community and bear aesthetics.

We had the opportunity to test and discuss ideas about age-discrepant relationships with a sample of ten members of the bear community, who considered themselves as 'silver daddies' or 'silver bears', and 15 young 'hunters' of silver daddies and bears. The interviews were conducted in Argentina through the Club de Osos de Buenos Aires (Bear Club of Buenos Aires) and the specialised website Growler for bears and hunters.

The responses of the silver daddies and bears confirm the importance of age, with an important presence of older people in the bear community. That community represents a space of freedom, in which age is not a barrier for social and sexual relationships: 'Nobody cares about your age' was an idea that frequently arises among bears, while one participant went a step further: 'If you are with a younger couple, silver daddies are just one more member of the group'.

Being a silver daddy involves perceiving themselves as being an object of desire for younger people, which contrasts with the position of older people in conventional gay communities. For instance, one interviewee asked: 'If you are a regular gay, you're older when you're 30. But if you're a sugar daddy, you're respected among the bears, older people are deemed to be interesting?', while, in a similar tone, others claimed: 'Gay saunas are catwalks … but here you are free, there's no age discrimination'. Being desired is related to a feeling of plenitude, as one of them mentioned: 'Being desired is an extremely pleasurable feeling. I don't feel ashamed of being who I am. I feel free and grateful for having found a younger couple'.

Despite this, rarely did the bears interviewed attribute the desire they arouse in their younger partners to a desire for the old. In most cases, such desire is associated with financial protection, 'They want your money. They want you for finding a job or for living on you', one said harshly), but also qualities they miss, such as security, lack of attachment or fulfillment of a parental role. For instance, one of them declared: 'They want to replace the image of a father who they never had', and another one that, 'I suppose they look for protection, someone who can guide them. Even if they welcome financial security, they also wish for affection'.

The responses of the young 'hunters' showed that they valued personal characteristics of bears, such as their confidence, care, acceptance, experience or guidance. Maturity is the metaphor that seems to organise the achievement associated with the passage of time, as well as a permanent reference to older bears. Younger partners talk in admiring terms about their masculinity, their experience, and their capacity to provide protection and care, in a relationship that involves mentorship and support, as well as empathy, confidence, and calm: 'I like them for their stability. I feel comfortable talking with him about serious topics, life and work issues, things that are important for older people. He takes into account my feelings'. In contrast, their young peers can be defined as, 'too focused on partying and having fun', or 'too ego-oriented'.

Beyond such personal characteristics, young gay males can also find sexual elements in silver bears. Maybe they are not so 'beautiful', but they are more sensual and seductive: white hair, hairy looks, elegance or charm are frequently mentioned. For instance, one of them said, 'I like white hair, broad hands, hairy chest, big bellies … white hair turns me on!', while another declared, 'I used to seek a stereotype of the perfect man, but now I'm not interested in perfection, and I prefer a way of behaving, a charming masculinity … I would choose a round belly rather than a pretty face'.

Obviously, the attracting traits of silver bears are also worth mentioning regarding sexuality and sexual relationships. Bears' calm, experience or affection seems to make sexual relationships richer. For example, one interviewee said: 'An older guy is not as basic as a younger one, he can be more affectionate, more playful, with less urgency to put his dick inside'). Such young gay men highlight relationships less focused on external beauty and appearance and based more on ways of touching, on body sensations, and sometimes involving a strong, if not disturbing attraction. Sexual relationships are not defined in confrontational terms: 'Being passive with a bigger guy who is not young any more, that feeling of being possessed by him … then I feel that my desire grows and that he also likes me because I'm younger. Sexual relationships with people of my age are more a fight for power'. As this excerpt exemplifies, relationships with bears eliminate rivalry and open up the possibility of a protection as the quality defining the bond.

Despite this, when asked, young gay men still put age limits to their sexual partners. Most of them spoke of an upper limit of 60 years old, and that number is associated with being physically fit, being active, and keeping a good (although not stereotypically conventional) appearance. However, it was surprising that many of the bears with whom they relate are in their seventies.

Finally here, it is also remarkable that many of the young 'bear hunters' expressed difficulty in telling their friends of their interests in 'silver daddies' and 'bears', which shows the workings of ageism in that they are fully aware of how unconventional such relationships are and anticipate a lack of understanding or even rejection from their same-age peers.

Pornography and alternative aesthetics of eroticism in later life

Alternative aesthetics of eroticising older bodies also appear in pornography. That may be surprising, since pornography has traditionally been considered the realm of youthful, sculpted, immaculate bodies. It sets a stage in which their protagonists (and particularly men) are always ready for endless sex sessions, many times performed in anonymous, emotionless and stereotyped ways (Fox and Bale, 2018). That is, pornography has helped to set a narrow youth-oriented sexual and erotic model of sexual relationships in which ageing and/or signs of infirmity do not seem to have a place.

However, the emergence of the internet and the turn of the porn business to digital platforms (Attwood, 2010) has opened new possibilities for including alternative models of erotic bodies. Such diversity also includes age diversity, and consequently, older people (and older bodies) have started to appear in sexualised ways among internet porn videos, being ready and easily accessible for wider younger and older audiences. Digital porn, as well allowing the consumption of professional videos casting older people, also permit older amateurs to produce their own video clips: it is as easy as turning on a webcam or digital video recorder, performing for the camera and uploading the result to massive porn hub websites (Ruberg, 2016).

In an interesting study, Zecca (2021) identified four sub-genres or ways of representing older people in contemporary pornography. The first one, labelled 'granny porn', casts mainly older women, who show clearly old bodies, stressing the presence of wrinkles, flaccid skin, sagging breasts, and other indicators of old age. In such videos, women are dependent on their younger (man) counterparts, and they are subjected to what Smith (2014) calls the 'enfreakment' process: old external signs are defined as 'abnormal', transforming the sexual scene to excessive, shocking and grotesque, which may attract certain market niches liking such 'eroticisation of abnormality'.

The second sub-genre is called 'grandpa porn' and depicts older men having sex with younger (apparently teenage) women. As in the previous sub-genre, 'old' features of men are also emphasised, but the meanings attached to older protagonists have nothing to do with dependency or abnormality, but with power: the videos show how men reaffirm their masculinity, imposing their sexual power over young, passive women, contradicting or overcompensating the cultural assumptions about age.

The 'stepmom porn' is a third sub-genre depicting ageing bodies. Unlike the previous sub-genres, this is more popular and included in the mainstream porn offer. Such videos show beautiful mature women, reminiscent of the MILF stereotype already discussed. In these videos, female performers are portrayed as active and agentic regarding sex, and they tend to be the ones that initiate the sexual activity (Ortiz and Tomson, 2017), many times with naïve young men (sometimes cast as their 'stepson', a neighbour or a friend of their son). Age differences between partners are evident, but unlike previous sub-genres, age markers are not stressed. Mature women are signified as wise and as using their ageless body to teach and sexually initiate their younger, inexpert counterpart. Such mature women can be depicted as self-confident, powerful, and seductive, defying traditional gender roles for heterosexual encounters, which may be the key to their sexual attractiveness (Vannier et al, 2014).

The four sub-genres include porn material mainly recorded by amateur older people, in which they exhibit themselves in ordinary sexual behaviour, many times as a part of a personal project of self-expression. In these videos, older people, and their older bodies, are presented without the stereotyped plots that characterise the previous sub-genres, in a more free space in which older bodies are shown as a legitimate object of desire.

As we can see, porn gives multiple, and sometimes contradictory, ways to resexualise older bodies. Some of them take advantage of the Western traditional view of older people (infirmity, ugliness, sexlessness), exaggerating them and transforming such bodies into 'freak' objects of desire. In other cases, such traditional views are also taken into account but in an opposite direction, 'exorcising' them by keeping an inner masculine power immune to negative external signs of age. Sometimes, such traditional versions are simply denied or ignored, and physical signs of age are minimised, while psychological attributes, such as sexual wisdom, are emphasised to construct a viable erotic of feminine older age. Age differences and open rupture with cultural norms regarding what is 'allowed', or even, in some cases, what should be 'disgusting' or 'unattractive', are apparently key to erotic arousal since, as Paasonen (2011, 2021) affirms, in porn, what is disgusting or forbidden often also arouses, excites and fascinates.

Looking beyond stereotypes, grassroots porn productions allow for expressing a truly alternative aesthetic eroticism in older age, one in which older people are shown as they are, affirming their value as erotic beings, capable of desire and being desired. It is in this way that such movement, if it spreads and reaches the mainstream culture, could be revolutionary, a real alternative to the traditional aesthetic of older age eroticism, far from both traditional models of decrepitude and ugliness and new models of sexy youthful, and active older adults.

Conclusion

In this chapter we have tried to explore the possibilities of developing an alternative aesthetic of eroticism in later life, an aesthetic that allows older people not just to express their sexual desire, but to also be considered as objects of desire for people of any age, including young people. We have described some examples coming from heterosexual relationships (such as sugar daddies, DILFs, cougars, or MILFs), from homosexual relationships (for example, silver bears), and in some porn sub-genres.

We have discussed how difficult it is to find such new aesthetics of eroticism when the traditional image of older people is associated with an asexual life marked by infirmities, decrepitude, and a body considered as 'ugly' taking into account contemporary youth-oriented standards of beauty. Sometimes these challenges are overcome by disembodying older people, emphasising qualities that are not just immune to the passage of time, but boosted by it: experience, maturity, or charm are qualities that could be found erotic in older people. Another way of re-sexualising older people is to extend the traditional youth-oriented models of beauty beyond young adulthood, and embracing just the opposite to dependant and infirm later life: a 'youthful ageing' in which success is defined as keeping younger qualities, including an 'ageless' body, to appear sexy regardless of age. The stereotype of MILFs is an epitome of such a strategy.

However, both ways of creating new aesthetics of eroticism in later life have a limit: they are probably more adequate for middle-aged adults than for older adults and, in the case of 'youthful ageing', could even function as a form of consolidating a cultural aversion to ageing. In fact, the only viable aesthetics of eroticism in later life identified in this chapter comes from niches far away from the mainstream: the silver bears in the case of gay culture, some forms of grassroots self-exposure in the case of porn.

Our analysis has shown how the intersection between age and gender is key to understanding the possibilities and constraints for an aesthetic of eroticism in later life. Aging is a gendered experience, from both an individual and social point of view. Thus, compared to their masculine counterparts, older women seem to have particular difficulties to find ways to be seen as objects of desire without showing a youthful appearance. In the case of homosexual persons, the 'gender gap' is still more marked: while we find literature exploring alternative aesthetics of older gay men in which age has a salient role, studies on aesthetics of eroticism in the case of older lesbian women or transsexual people are virtually absent. Without a doubt, this is a major gap if we want to have complete and inclusive knowledge of the field.

Also, we must consider the production of sexual possibilities of our later capitalism in an ageing society. To sell products, lifestyles and even desires to a greater public and with a postmodern culture that makes irrelevant the differences of age (Neugarten, 1992; Katz, 1996). But this openness couldn't be reduced to a market logic. The deep democratisation of societies moves to the acceptance of sexual possibilities. The movement for diversity allows the institutionalisation of different sexual orientations and identities, that is a real novelty in Western history.

New ways of re-sexualising older age, despite the difficulties they face in emerging, may challenge traditional views of ageing and sexuality. We should be attentive to their evolution, particularly to the possibility of such ways of re-sexualising older people to transcend the marginal position they occupy now, and be able to be included in a broad sexual imaginary.

References

Alarie, M. (2019) 'They're the ones chasing the cougar': relationship formation in the context of age-hypogamous intimate relationships, *Gender & Society*, 33(3): 463–85.

Alarie, M. (2020) Sleeping with younger men: women's accounts of sexual interplay in age-hypogamous intimate relationships, *The Journal of Sex Research*, 57(3): 322–34.

Antfolk, J., Salo, B., Alanko, K., Bergen, E., Corander, J., Sandnabba, N.K. and Santtila, P. (2015) Women's and men's sexual preferences and activities with respect to the partner's age: Evidence for female choice, *Evolution and Human Behavior*, 36: 73–9.

Attwood, F. (ed) (2010) *Porn.com: Making Sense of Online Pornography*, Peter Lang.

Berardo, F.M., Appel, J. and Berardo, D.H. (1993) Age dissimilar marriages: Review and assessment,*Journal of Aging Studies*, 7: 93–106.

Bergström, M. and Kramer, R. (2015) Gendered attitudes to age on online dating sites (France, 2000s), *Clio: Women, Gender, History*, 42(2): 125–46.

Clarke, L.H. (2010) *Facing Age: Women Growing Older in Anti-aging Culture*, Rowman & Littlefield Publishers.

Clarke, L.H. (2018) Women, aging, and beauty culture: navigating the social perils of looking old, *Generations*, 41(4): 104–8.

Collard, R.C. (2012) Cougar figures, gender and the performances of predation, *Gender, Place & Culture*, 19(4): 518–40.

Collisson, B. and Ponce de Leon, L. (2020) Perceived inequity predicts prejudice towards age-gap relationships, *Current Psychology*, 39 : 2108–15.

Coupland, J. (2009) Discourse, identity and change in mid-to-late life: interdisciplinary perspectives on language and ageing, *Ageing and Society*, 29: 849–61.

Daly, S.E. (2017) *Sugar Babies and Sugar Daddies: An Exploration of Sugar Dating on Canadian Campuses* (Doctoral dissertation, Carleton University).

Drummond, M.J. (2010) Younger and older gay men's bodies, *Gay and Lesbian Issues and Psychology Review*, 6: 31–41.

Ferrero Camoletto, R. (2019) Questioning the sexy oldie: masculinity, age and sexuality in the Viagra era, in A. King, K. Almack and R.L. Jones (eds) *Intersections of Ageing, Gender, and Sexualities*, Policy Press: pp 209–22.

Fox, N.J. and Bale, C. (2018) Bodies, pornography and the circumscription of sexuality: a new materialist study of young people's sexual practices, *Sexualities*, 21(3): 393–409.

Friedman, M. (2014) Beyond MILF: exploring sexuality and feminism in public motherhood, *Atlantis*, 36(2): 49–60.

García-Sierra, G. (2019) *Diccionario Filosófico* (2nd edn), Biblioteca de Filosofía en Español.

Gewirtz-Meydan, A., Hafford-Letchfield, T., Benyamini, Y., Phelan, A., Jackson, J. and Ayalon, L. (2018) Ageism and sexuality, in *Contemporary Perspectives on Ageism*, Springer, pp 199–62.

Giuliani, G. (2020) *Who is Older? Gender and Age Differences in Heterosexual Couples* (Doctoral dissertation, European University Institute).

Gobind, J. and Du Plessis, G. (2015) Sugar daddy: the student attraction, *Gender and Behaviour*, 13(2): 6720–9.

González, C. (2007) Age-graded sexualities: the struggles of our ageing body, *Sexuality & Culture*, 11: 31–47.

Gough, B. and Flanders, G. (2009) Celebrating 'obese' bodies: gay' bears' talk about weight, body image and health, *International Journal of Men's Health*, 8(3): 235–53.

Gustafson, P. and Fransson, U. (2015) Age differences between spouses: sociodemographic variation and selection, *Marriage & Family Review*, 51: 610–32.

Hennen, P. (2005) Bear bodies, bear masculinity: recuperation, resistance, or retreat? *Gender and Society*, 19: 25–43.

Hillman, J. (2012) *Sexuality and Aging: Clinical Perspectives*, Springer.

Hinchliff, S. and Gott, M. (2017) Ageing and sexuality in western societies: changing perspectives on sexual activity, sexual expression and the 'sexy' older body, in R. Harding and E. Peel (eds) *Ageing and Sexualities*, Routledge, pp 11–31.

Iacub, R. (2006) *Erótica y Vejez. Perspectivas de Occidente*, Paidós.

Iacub, R. and Villar, F. (2021) The aesthetic(s) of eroticism in later life, in P. Simpson, P. Reynolds and T. Hafford-Letchfield (eds), *Desexualisation in Later Life: The Limits of Sex and Intimacy*, Policy Press, pp 53–75.

Kaklamanidou, B. (2012) Pride and prejudice: celebrity versus fictional cougars, *Celebrity Studies*, 3(1): 78–89.

Katz, S. (1996) *Disciplining Old Age: The Formation of Gerontological Knowledge*, University Press Virginia.

Kaufman, G. and Chin Phua, V. (2003) Is ageism alive in date selection among men? Age requests among gay and straight men in internet personal ads, *Journal of Men's Studies*, 11: 225–35.

Manley, E., Levitt, H. and Mosher, C. (2007) Understanding the bear movement in gay male culture: redefining masculinity, *Journal of Homosexuality*, 53(4): 89–112.

Marshall, B. (2010) Science, medicine and virility surveillance: 'sexy seniors' in the pharmaceutical imagination, *Sociology of Health and Illness*, 32: 211–24.

McKenzie, L. (2015) *Age-Dissimilar Couples and Romantic Relationships: Ageless Love?* Palgrave Macmillan.

Montemurro, B. and Siefken, J.M. (2012) MILFs and matrons: images and realities of mothers' sexuality, *Sexuality & Culture*, 16(4): 366–88.

Montemurro, B. and Siefken, J.M. (2014) Cougars on the prowl? New perceptions of older women's sexuality, *Journal of Aging Studies*, 28: 35–43.

Neugarten, B. (1992) *Los Significados de la Edad*, Herder.

Ortiz, R.R. and Thomson, B. (2017) Content effects: pornography and sexually explicit content, in P. Rossler (ed) *The International Encyclopedia of Media Effects*, John Wiley & Sons, pp 246–57.

Oswald, F., Hughes, S., Champion, A. and Pedersen, C.L. (2020) In search of the appeal of the 'DILF', *Psychology & Sexuality*, 1–19.

Paasonen, S. (2011) *Carnal Resonance: Affect and Online Pornography*, MIT Press.

Paasonen, S. (2021) 'Old dirty pops and hot chicks': age differences in pornographic fantasies, in C. M. Scarcelli, D. Chronaki, S. de Vuyst, and S. Villanueva (eds) *Gender and Sexuality in the European Media*, Routledge, pp 146–60.

Quidley-Rodriguez, N. and De Santis, J.P. (2019) A concept analysis of bear identity, *Journal of Homosexuality*, 66(1): 60–76.

Rowe, J.W. and Kahn, R.L. (2015) Successful aging 2.0: conceptual expansions for the 21st century, *The Journals of Gerontology: Series B*, 70(4): 593–96.

Ruberg, B. (2016) Doing it for free: digital labour and the fantasy of amateur online pornography, *Porn Studies*, 3(2): 147–59.

Sandberg, L. (2016) In lust we trust? Masculinity and sexual desire in later life, *Men and Masculinities*, 19: 192–208.

Settersten, R.A., Jr. and Trauten, M. (2008) The new terrain of old age: hallmarks, freedoms, and risks, in V. Bengtson, M. Silverstein, D. Putney and S. Gans (eds) *Handbook of Theories of Aging*, Springer Publishing Company, pp 455–69.

Silva, T. (2019) 'Daddies', 'cougars', and their partners past midlife: gender attitudes and relationship and sexual well-being among older adults in age-heterogenous partnerships, *Socius*, 5: 1–15.

Slevin, K.F. and Linneman, T.J. (2010) Old gay men's bodies and masculinities, *Men and Masculinities*, 12: 483–507.

Smith, A. (2018) Bulging biceps and tender kisses: the sexualisation of fatherhood, *Social Semiotics*, 28(3): 315–29.

Smith, C. (2014) 'It's important that you don't smell a suit on this stuff': aesthetics and politics in alt porn, in E. Biasin, G. Maina and F. Zecca (eds) *Porn after Porn: Contemporary Alternative Pornographies*, Mimesis International, pp 57–83.

Smith, L., Yang, L., Veronese, N., Soysal, P., Stubbs, B. and Jackson, S.E. (2019) Sexual activity is associated with greater enjoyment of life in older adults, *Sexual Medicine*, 7(1): 11–18.

Smith, T.W. (2011) *Cross-National Differences in Attitudes towards Homosexuality*, NORC/University of Chicago GSS Cross-national Report, No. 31.

Sontag, S. (1997) The double standard of aging, in M. Pearsall (ed) *The Other within Us: Feminist Explorations of Women and Aging*, Westview Press.

Suen, Y-T. (2017) Older single gay men's body talk: resisting and rigidifying the aging discourse in the gay community, *Journal of Homosexuality*, 64(3): 397–414.

Syme, M.L. and Cohn, T.J. (2016) Examining aging sexual stigma attitudes among adults by gender, age, and generational status, *Aging & Mental Health*, 20: 36–45.

Van Bauwel, S. (2021) Invisible aged femininities in popular culture: representational strategies deconstructed, in C. M. Scarcelli, D. Chronaki, S. de Vuyst and S. Villanueva (eds), *Gender and Sexuality in the European Media*, Routledge, pp 135–45.

Vanderheiden, E. (2025) 'A matter of age?' Love relationships between older women and younger men: the so-called 'cougar' phenomenon, in C.-H. Mayer and E. Vanderheiden (eds) *International Handbook of Love*, Springer, pp 369–90.

Vannier, S.A., Currie, A.B. and O'Sullivan, L.F. (2014) Schoolgirls and soccer moms: a content analysis of free 'teen' and 'MILF' online pornography, *The Journal of Sex Research*, 51(3): 253–64.

Vares, T. (2009) Reading the 'sexy oldie': gender, age(ing) and embodiment, *Sexualities*, 12(4): 503–24.

Villar, F., Serrat, R., de Sao José, J.M., Montero, M., Arias, C.J., Nina-Estrella, R., Curcio, C-L, de Oliveira, R., Tirro, V. and Alfonso, A. (2019) Age-discrepant couples involving an older adult: the final frontier of ageism? Attitudes in eight Latin American countries, *Journal of Intergenerational Relationships*, 17(4): 430–48.

Widmer, E., Ritschard, G. and Muller, N. (2009) The de-standardization of the life course: are men and women equal? *Advances in Life Course Research*, 14: 28–39.

World Health Organization (2002) *Active Ageing: A Policy Framework* (No. WHO/NMH/NPH/02.8), World Health Organization.

Zecca, F. (2021) No country for old men? Representations of the ageing body in contemporary pornography, in C.M. Scarcelli, D. Chronaki, S. de Vuyst and S. Villanueva (eds) *Gender and Sexuality in the European Media*, Routledge, pp 190–202.

3

Older swinging, 'casual' intimacies and sex outside coupledom

Eir-Anne Edgar

Introduction

This chapter begins with a review of studies that examine the gendered, sexual stereotypes of older people in contrast to the diversity of lived ageing people's sexual lives. While the focus of this chapter is on non-monogamy and ageing people, both academic studies and filmic portrayals on this topic are scant. In the process of locating portrayals for analysis, indie-produced pornography and educational films for gerontology students offered some of the most diverse portrayals of non-monogamous ageing people. However, these films are difficult to locate and expensive to obtain. Instead, this chapter analyses three independently produced films that offer accessibility via streaming services (such as Amazon Prime and Netflix). Each film addresses different issues associated with non-monogamy and ageing people. The German film *Cloud 9* (2008) portrays the casual sexuality of 67-year-old Inge and illustrates how desire and intimacy can take on many forms. Canadian queer film *Gerontophilia* (2014) also upsets stereotypes of ageing sexuality and illustrates attraction between older and younger men. *Boynton Beach Club* (2005) offers a dynamic depiction of the lives of older people; the film's financial success should not come as a surprise to those who have seen it. As well, this chapter includes a brief analysis of the Nancy Myers film trailer for *It's Complicated*, (2009) a movie that epitomises Hollywood's approach to ageing people and sexuality. Despite the dynamic portrait of ageing people and non-monogamy that scholarly studies are beginning to document, filmic portrayals have only recently begun to move beyond stereotypes about ageing people and their sexual lives, underscoring the importance of supporting alternative and diverse film and other media. Culture has the power to effect change, and more diverse representations of ageing people and non-monogamy in film and other texts can impact society and policy, for the better.

Representing data, representing age

Sex is a key component in many ageing people's lives. However, older people are stereotyped and/or infantilised in culture. This affects depictions of ageing people in film and television, which features portrayals of people as too old or too infirm to have sex lives. While this may be true for some individuals, many studies indicate that older people are interested in sex and, in fact, have healthy and vibrant sex lives. One issue is defining what qualifies as old age, as people have begun to live longer and healthier lives than before, while at the same time, the Hollywood requirements for old get lower. As noted in this volume's introduction, after age 50 and into the sixth decade, older people 'experience a process of de-eroticisation'. However, Hollywood standards sometimes place actors aged 45 and older within the framework of elder, particularly in the case of women. Perhaps not so surprising, studies also find that older adults are often sexually active:

> In a study of Americans over the age of 60, researchers found that 66% of women said sex was an important part of their relationships with their husbands and that 70% of sexually active women were either 'as satisfied or even more satisfied with their sexual lives than they were in their forties'. (Kingsberg, 2002: 432, cited in Montemurro and Chewning, 2017: 1)

Not only are older individuals having sex, but they are also having pleasurable sex, despite the existing representations. Sexually active older people are often depicted in film and television as comedic, portrayals play on ageing people 'as not sexually desirable, not sexually desirous and not sexually capable' (Vares, 2009: 503).

Contemporary representations of older people rarely portray individuals as being interested in or able to have sex. Films that do feature portrayals of sex often rely on stereotypes. Some of these stereotypes stem from an aversion to depictions of ageing, as sexuality is often synonymous with youthfulness. Other stereotypes are gendered. Allen and Roberto note:

> Older people who speak about their sexuality often are viewed either as exaggerating or as deviant – evidenced in the term *dirty old man* – or are called *cute* when they express physical affection for one another … Misinformation about age-related physiological changes and chronic disease also contributes to the myths surrounding sexuality in late life. (2009: 14)

Few adults wish to be portrayed as dirty or cute when it comes to their sexual lives, though many films rely on these tropes. Still other representations focus on disorders when it comes to older people and sex. Bouman and Kleinplatz note:

> much of the literature on sexuality in older people focuses on sexual problems, leaving clinicians with the impression that older adults have either dismal or non-existent sex lives. Sex is assumed to be for the young, beautiful, able-bodied, and heterosexual. Older people are often perceived and portrayed as post-sexual. Unfortunately, the result of these negative perceptions is that older people themselves often hold similar self-stereotypes. (2015: 1)

Even when older people are portrayed as sexually active, these portrayals are few and far between. Lauzen and Dozier note that the few representations of older people in film do not reflect the reality of a sizeable, ageing population. To illustrate this, they note that:

> representation of women 60 and older was 14 points below the US populations figures. Representation of men 60 and older was ten points below the US population. As these percentages indicate, popular films favor male characters in their 30s and 40s and female characters in their 20s and 30s. These findings confirm that larger portions of female characters continue to be younger than their male counterparts. (2005: 437)

Not only are filmic representations of ageing people rare, but these representations are also not very diverse.

Representations of sexy seniors tend to be heterosexual, white, cisgendered, and monogamous, and this homogeneity can have serious negative effects. Bouman and Kleinplatz find that many older people do not fit within these narrow parameters. They highlight the realities that, 'many older people considered exploring more diverse and alternative forms of dating and relationship formation' (2015: 1). In a review of gerontological literature, Kristin Scherrer finds that representation is important for understanding and advocacy. She notes, for example:

> that heterosexual relationships and penile-vaginal sexual behaviors might be more likely to receive support than same-sex relationships and behaviors, but further research is needed in this area. Knowing that the sexualities of older adults are enabled and constrained will additionally enable care facilities to craft policy that supports both same-sex and heterosexual relationships and behaviors. (2009: 5)

In addition to specific representations of older people and sexuality being dominant in filmic portrayals, we also see gendered representations of older sex that can have negative impacts.

Older women are often portrayed as sexless in films, despite data that indicates otherwise. In an analysis of Swedish films, Bildtgard finds that the 'gendered double-standard of ageing is at work in all nine films with elderly women portrayed less often than sexually active elderly men and the usual sexual combination being that of an elderly man and a younger woman – with no examples of the opposite situation' (cited in Vares, 2009: 504). In discussing US films, Montemurro and Chewning find 'the lack of public images of older women's sexuality and desirability, particularly unmarried or unpartnered older women, contributes to their cultural invisibility and reinforces a narrative of ageing as sexual decline' (2017: 127). Despite the limited representations of older women and sexuality in films, Allen and Roberto claim that older women *are* sexual. 'The overwhelming response from both female (95%) and male (93%) students was the acknowledgment that contrary to stereotypes – and, thus, expectations – older women still feel sexual in their later years' (2009: 13).

Representing reality

Not only are older men and women having sex, despite limited representations in films, they are having non-monogamous sex. Many filmic depictions re-centre monogamy and the marriage structure. In a key study, Bouman and Kleinpatz (2015: 2) discuss how older people consider sexuality outside of the marriage structure. They write:

> In previous studies, older people discussed the importance of looking for relationships that are based on emotional and sexual equality, but not necessarily on cohabitation or monogamy. Many older widows were opposed to remarriage or considered it impossible … They often associated dating with loss of independence because the men they dated wanted marriage … They expressed concern that a potential remarriage might entail an unequal division of labour … In contrast, they associated widowhood with freedom. They enjoyed what they termed their 'selfish' abilities to do what they wanted … As a result, widows were more open to experimenting with different forms of relationship without cohabitation … In some cases, they made the effort to separate emotional closeness, physical proximity and geographical distance.

Not only do these findings upset traditional forms of heteronormative monogamy, as well as stereotypical understandings of gender, sexuality, and older people, they also reflect recent data that shows non-monogamous practices to be widespread. Rubin et al write 'A 2002 representative sample of adults from National Survey of Family Growth (NSFG) found that approximately 18% of women and 23% of men were engaged in non-monogamy … These percentages suggest that an estimated 19 million Americans participate in non-monogamy' (2014: 19).

Non-academic publications that *do* discuss non-monogamy and sex tread a careful line, one that continues to place monogamous marriage at the centre of our understanding of older people and sexuality. In a piece for *Psychology Today*, a website that invites 'luminaries in the field of psychology to write about their own work and that of others in a way that is accessible to lay readers', Elisabeth Sheff (2017) writes about ageing in polyamorous families. She states:

> Like many others in their 60s and 70s, these polyamorous folks expressed a decreasing focus on sex. Many of them still enjoy sex and maintain ongoing sexual relationships with multiple partners, sometimes using common techniques to sustain those sex lives, such as taking Viagra, setting the stage carefully, having kinds of sex that do not center around genital penetration, and making sure the timing is right. A small minority of women declared themselves done with sex completely, or at least for their foreseeable future. Several relationships had transitioned from sexual to platonic, with affection and cuddling but no sex. In most of those cases, the older poly folks still had sex – just not with that long-term partner. The lack of sexual connection did not seem to damage the relationships, and some were incredibly close and durable through the transition from sexual to platonic.

Sheff emphasises the relatability of 'these polyamorous folks', utilising several aforementioned stereotypes about older people and sex (decreased desire for sex in general, erectile dysfunction, sexless women). Despite Sheff's inclusion of stereotypes about older people and their sexual lives, there is some data that *is* interesting, yet unexplored in this piece – older people with multiple sex partners, non-penetrative sex, and multiple sexual partners are all underrepresented in both studies and portrayals of older people and sexuality. In another piece for the website publication of long running magazine *Good Housekeeping*, Elizabeth Durand Streisand discusses a mid-fifties couple in her article 'We're a senior couple who swings with other seniors'. Similarly to Sheff's approach of emphasising the couple's relatability factor, she narrates:

> Mark and Deanna, both in their mid-fifties, got married 5 years ago. Neither has children from any prior relationships. They live in Las Vegas, Nevada, where they enjoy walking their dogs, doing puzzles, and seeing new movies on date nights. They also like going to places like The Green Door, a nearby night club that hosts various swingers' parties. To this couple, casual sex with strangers is a recreational activity just like any other. (2016)

For the remainder of the article, Streisand relays the couple's experiences of swinging and the rules that guide their swinging (such as always discussing things as a couple). Like Sheff's article, this piece strikes a balance between discussing an underrepresented population, while also emphasising their relatability – swinging is 'a recreational activity just like any other' (although, this note makes one very curious about Streisand's waterskiing or hiking practices, as far as 'recreational activities' go!).

Existing data on non-monogamy and ageing people is limited but reveals some insights about both gender and queerness when it comes to sex. Suen writes about older single gay men and dating. Their study states:

> some participants saw the lack of a regular partner as a downside of being single, many others saw being single as giving them greater freedom for sexual exploration. Patrick, for example, said being single allowed him to have multiple sex partners. He said that he was not interested in having sex with the same man too frequently, no matter how attractive he might be. (2015: 143)

In another study, Malta and Farquharsen discuss older people and sexual relationships. They find:

> Overall, the research into dating and courtship in late life suggests there is a strong desire among older adults – especially women – to retain their independence and maintain separate lives from their romantic partners. The studies discussed above suggest that late-life couples want to maintain close, romantic and intimate relationships while living separately – a phenomenon which has since become known as living-apart-together (LAT). (2012: 237)

Many of the older people interviewed for their study relished the LAT relationships they established,

> Like Stewart and Nigel and their non-monogamous arrangements, the relationships were negotiated but they did not appear disposable … Dating services, in particular online dating, gave these older adults the means to be able to pursue this ideal by allowing them access to many more potential partners than would otherwise be available. (2012: 241)

In these few studies, older people express a reluctance to re-couple simply for the purposes of being in a couple structure and they are interested in (and are having) an active and varied sex life.

Further data illustrates that baby boomers are interested in sexual experimentation. Rowntree's excellent study, 'The influence of ageing on baby boomers' not so straight sexualities' further illustrates how the typical filmic portrayals of older people and corresponding sexual stereotypes are inaccurate. Rowntree (2015: 980) writes:

> In this study, later life is found to be a prime time that these non-exclusive baby boomers explore, experiment or reappraise their sexual orientations or preferences. Yet the agency of baby boomers to express their sexuality differently in their senior years appears mediated by relationship status, with those no longer in long-established heterosexual relationships more likely to challenge hetero-normative arrangements. The study shows women in this subset to be particularly open to the possibility of future sexual relationships with women, pointing to possible differences on the basis of gender. These findings are consistent with recent research that shows sexual expression to be more dynamic, changeable over time and responsive to social contexts, particularly for women.

Like the studies that illustrate that older widowed women have a propensity to favor the LAT (living apart together) relationship over the marriage structure, Rowntree's work finds that older women are also more interested in experimenting with their sexuality. This data also works to unsettle the staid stereotypes of sexless older women as portrayed in film.

Despite the openness and variation of older peoples' sexual experiences as highlighted via the various studies, filmic portrayals utilise many stereotypes, yet also offer some diverse representations. In the sections that follow, analyses of a film trailer and three films discusses issues of gendered stereotypes, reconfigurations of monogamy, reformulations of intimacy and desire, infantilisation of older people, portrayals of nude older bodies, and the reversals of queer stereotypes. The films deploy some stereotypes, yet also offer vibrant portrayals of resexualisation and older people.

It's Complicated

In the 2009 Nancy Myers film trailer for *It's Complicated*, Meryl Streep confides in her friends that she is having an affair with a married man. Only, the married man is her ex-husband, played by Alec Baldwin. At the same time, the trailer indicates that Streep's character is also dating Adam, her architect, played by Steve Martin. The trailer is sexy, fun, and a bit risqué. However, the film is not exactly the triangle of intrigue and sex that the trailer makes it out to be. While Streep *is* sleeping with her ex-husband (now married to the woman he cheated on Streep with during their marriage), she is not sleeping with or even in a relationship with Martin's character. Instead, Martin realises that Streep is having a fling with her ex and tells her that her situation is too complicated for him. When

Streep finally sorts things out with Baldwin (and ends the affair), she must convince Martin/Adam that she is single and that she only wants to date him. Although the trailer presents a sexy film premise, one featuring Meryl Streep having sex with multiple men and the envy of her friends, the movie is far *less* complicated than the title promises – rather than an exploration of non-monogamy, we instead see the marriage relationship resituated (via Streep and Baldwin's rekindling) and then, presumably, monogamy between Streep and Martin, though there is never a sex scene depicted, as the film ends when their relationship begins. The 'sexy senior' film is a prevalent formula in Hollywood. Films like *Something's Gotta Give*, *Book Club* and *Because I Said So* depict Meryl Streep, Diane Keaton and other ageing Hollywood greats as women who are interested in sex, yet not often having very much of it. On the other hand, older male actors (such as Jack Nicholson in *Something's Gotta Give*) are having sex, with young, attractive twentysomething women. However, eventually these men settle down and pair off with a more age-appropriate woman. Just as these films re-situate monogamous marital structures, they also re-situate stereotypes of men – Nicholson can age, date, and have sex with younger women, but it isn't until Diane Keaton's character attracts the affections of a younger Keanu Reeves that she catches Nicholson's eye. Men are also allowed to visibly age on the screen in a way that women are not.

Cloud 9

German film, *Cloud 9* (*Wolke 9*), portrays ageing sexuality with nude, lusty sex scenes. Inge, 67 years old and married to Werner for over 30 years, has an affair with Karl. Before the title page appears, viewers are treated to a nearly 10-minute-long scene in which Inge brings Karl the pants she has tailored for him. After trying them on in front of her, they are both overcome with desire, kissing, and touching on the carpeted floor. They have sex, and it is a fully nude scene, though Inge leaves her shirt on. Later, we see Inge bathing her husband Werner, and this scene of domestic care becomes very sexual, though it cuts to a new scene before viewers see it develop into sex. However, not long after this scene, the couple does have sex in front of the camera, and it is a fully nude scene for both actors. Repeatedly, *Cloud 9* depicts ageing sexuality – between Inge and 76-year-old Karl, and between Inge and husband Werner. As Roger Ebert notes, 'The director, Andreas Dresen, presents the sex scenes as if they involve two 20-year-olds, as she should. During sex, you have only two ages: immortal or dead' (2006: par. 7). There is also a scene in which Inge inspects her nude body in front of a mirror and in which she masturbates while in the bathtub. *Cloud 9* shows ageing bodies, bodies that are desired and that are desiring, and illustrates that sex is a key component of life for ageing individuals.

Interestingly, some scholars are guilty of stereotyping Inge, Werner and Karl as dissatisfied, though there is no evidence of this in the film. Liya Sun writes,

> Inge's eagerness to change her monotonous life is demonstrated in one scene where she carefully watches her nude reflection in a mirror, telling herself and the audience that she is still an attractive woman. Her shrivelled, wilted body is shown explicitly and naturally, but without the intention of evoking sexual arousal … Inge is addicted to the unethical relationship and is thrilled like never before. (2019: 205)

The scene in which Inge gazes at her nude body does not contain any dialogue. She merely runs her hands over her body in an appreciative way – it is neither 'shriveled' nor 'wrinkled' and whether it arouses sexual desire is up to the minds of viewers. Sun's reading of this scene generally reflects negative stereotyping of ageing bodies on film, even if those bodies are portrayed as desired and desiring. In discussing the same scene, film critic Roger Ebert (2009) writes, 'There is a scene where Inge stands naked in front of a mirror and looks at herself. Such a moment of honesty is common enough in the movies, but she does it for so long that our minds begin to supply her thoughts about the inexorable fading of youth.' However, Inge's very active sex life contradicts any notions of the 'fading of youth'.

Despite the pleasure that all three seemingly gain from their sexual situation, *Cloud 9* does not depict Inge as freely moving between the two men in the film. She feels guilty about her relationship with Karl, and despite the advice of her daughter Petra to keep the relationship a secret, she reveals the affair to Werner. She tells him, 'After living together for so long we should be able to talk to one another if something like this happens.' However, despite their long relationship and high level of regard for one another, Inge is forced to move in with Karl. She later tells Werner that they should separate. In this touching scene, Werner opens a bottle of wine, and they briefly reflect on their relationship. He says, 'I was often surprised by you in the past few weeks. You were like a young girl, now I know why.' He asks what he did wrong for her to be with Karl, and she says nothing. 'Otherwise, we couldn't have lived together for 30 years.' Later that night, Inge and Karl receive a phone call from Petra that Werner has died. Though we get no details about Werner's death, it is not difficult to imagine that the dissolution of their relationship has had some effect.

Cloud 9 has many steamy sex scenes, but also offers alternative forms of intimacy. The film contains little dialogue, but many scenes in which Inge is in close physical proximity to Karl and/or Werner. Brewing tea in the kitchen, listening to a record together, washing dishes, and other domestic scenes are charged with a sense of intimacy. In one sex scene, Karl is unable to maintain an erection. Despite this, Inge smiles and reclines on the bed, satisfied. He tells her a joke and she laughs and laughs – the scene reads as if the joke is an alternative form of intimacy from the sex they set out to have, yet telling and hearing the joke is as satisfying as sex. In this moment, viewers are presented with an alternative form of intimacy to sex. According to Linn Sandberg, intimacy and sex can change for men as they age. Sandberg writes,

> When it is no longer possible to have children and intercourse is no longer an option, intimacy surfaces as a fluid middle ground between the sexual and the non-sexual. Intimacy could be something sexual, it could involve fondling and lead to orgasms … If men are expected always to want to have sex and male sexuality is very much linked to the penis and the ability to perform during intercourse, a shift towards intimacy may in effect relieve some of the pressure on men. (2013: 261)

Further, couples who reach late middle age initially identify changes in their sexual lives negatively, but their perspective can shift as time goes by. Gewirtz-Meydan et al (2019) write, 'Midlife couples (ages 50–69) were distressed by changes in their sex lives likely because they impede couples from performing gendered sexuality … In contrast, later life couples (ages 70–86) were more likely to emphasise the importance of emotional intimacy over sex as they age' (2019: 293). *Cloud 9* portrays both physical and emotional intimacy between Inge, Werner and Karl, reflecting the findings from these studies.

As people age, prevalent stereotypes perpetuated via depictions in film and even in academic scholarship can negatively impact sexual identity. In a study investigating comedic films and the sexuality of older people, Gatling et al find:

> The discourse of ageing as disseminated by Hollywood may still pre-dominantly represent older people as celibate, monogamous and heterosexual but occasionally films are released that present a different view. Old age holds a multitude of fears for those people who are not yet there … To top it all off is the perception that ageing is accompanied by a loss of intimacy – one of the most basic human needs. (2017: 23)

Further, stereotypical portrayals can impact how ageing people feel about their sexual identity. Gewirtz-Meydan et al write,

> As older people encounter health issues that affect their sexual function, many adopt a wider definition of sexual activity. Social constraints and *the delegitimisation of their sexuality* affects their sense of autonomy and wellbeing and narrows their indicators of how successful they are in remaining sexual and/or expressing their sexuality. (2019: 295, emphasis added)

Films such as *Cloud 9* work to re-frame narrow portrayals of ageing people and sexuality and legitimise under- or misrepresented individuals.

Boynton Beach Club

Boynton Beach Club follows a small group of older people navigating a range of issues – recently widowed or divorced, returning to the dating pool, asserting independence, and even re-learning how to drive a car. Of the films analysed in this chapter, this film offers the most diverse depictions of ageing people, though at times it utilises stereotypes, and it only depicts heterosexual characters. The Boynton Beach Bereavement Club (referred to hereafter as BBBC) serves as a social group for single older people in the community. Although the film does not exclusively address sexuality, it is a central topic. Widower Jack joins the BBBC, where he meets self-proclaimed ladies' man Harry, who tells Jack, 'Women to men – it's an 8:1 ratio. I've never been so popular.' Jack, more than 3 months after his wife's death, still has her message on their answering machine. He meets Sandy at the BBBC, who is friendly and open. He finally takes her up on an invitation for a date but treats her as he would his former wife Phyllis – they go for an early bird Chinese buffet dinner, which she does not enjoy. When he apologises for talking so much about his wife while on their date, Sandy tells him that this means they must have had a good marriage, 'and if you had a good marriage, it means you're not afraid to enter a new relationship'. However, Sandy is not exactly as she seems. Though she tells Jack that she is widowed, they run into her ex-husband while out on a date. Her explanation to Jack is that after her husband left, she felt it was like a death and 'a lot of people are threatened by divorces. At least if you're a widow you get sympathy'. Though Jack and Sandy do finally have sex, it does not go smoothly. She shows him her breasts, and this partial nudity is the only scene with on-camera nudity in the film, though there are suggestive scenes of characters wrapped in towels and sheets. They do not initially have sex that evening, preferring (at Jack's nervous request) to cuddle. However, the morning sun brings forth a change, as Jack wakes up and looks at (presumably) his erect penis under the sheet. He leans over to kiss Sandy's shoulder, and though the camera fades to black, it is implied that they have had sex.

Though Harry claims to be a ladies' man, when he meets Florence from the internet for a real-life date, he chickens out. First, he finds her vibrators in the bathroom. Then, when he finds her lying in bed clad in sexy lingerie, he leaves (and leaves money on the dresser). He attempts to give Jack advice before a date night with Sandy, telling him that sex with someone who is not your wife is very different, you see her breasts and butt and 'it hits you – you're about to have sex with an old lady'. Though Jack tells him sex is not on the cards, Harry says, 'people think you get to a certain age and there's no more sex. That ain't true'. As a foil to nervous widower Jack, Harry is an overly self-assured impresario, with little evidence to justify his ego.

Erectile dysfunction is a stereotypical punchline in the film. Jack is embarrassed at a pharmacy when he purchases Viagra, and the pharmacist very loudly tells him about possible side effects. The older women nearby giggle and continue to do so when the pharmacist yells out the aisle number in which Jack can find condoms. And, at a BBBC meeting, one woman asks the group, 'What do you say to a fella who can't raise the flag?' Another woman answers with, 'forget him, find yourself a boy toy!' and the room explodes with laughter.

Companionship and independence are also themes. After Marty is killed in an accident, Marilyn's children bring her an unwanted dog, telling her 'it'll keep you company'. Her daughter Denise also wants her to move in with them, though this does not seem inviting (their accident-prone young boys are always screaming and breaking things in the background). At Marilyn's dismissal, Denise asserts that Marty did everything for her mother, including drive. Marilyn retorts that she will learn. Jack's daughter also expresses concern about his ability to make choices. Although his wife has been dead for over 3 months, she states that it is 'too soon for Gramps to have a lady friend' when she hears Sandy's voice on the answering machine.

Boynton Beach Club offers a mixed bag of representations of sexuality. While some harmful stereotypes serve as punchlines, like the emphasis on ageing bodies not so sexually desirable, other portrayals, such as widows' and widowers' navigation of dating life, illustrate dynamic and active sexuality in the lives of older people. Roger Ebert, in a review of the film writes,

> *Boynton Beach Club* is an indie teen sex comedy of the sort with which director Susan Seidelman began her career. The characters still worry about dating and learning to drive, buying condoms and getting naked, only now the teens are in their 60s and 70s, live in Florida instead of SoHo or the East Village, and use the Internet rather than newspapers to place their personals ads. (2006: par. 2)

Thinking about the film as a 'teen sex comedy', as Ebert suggests, helps us understand its successful depictions of older people. Although it plays upon stereotypes like erectile dysfunction for laughs, *Boynton Beach Club* portrays the resexualisation of older people in a successful and entertaining way.

Gerontophilia

Gerontophilia (see also Chapter 4) depicts Melvyn, an older man residing in an assisted living facility and his relationship with Lake, a young man working at the facility. This queer film reverses some stereotypes and depicts nudity (of the young and old) in both sexual and non-sexual settings. The movie follows Lake and traces his gradual recognition and acceptance of his burgeoning fetish for older men. Though he has a girlfriend who is also presumably his age (early twenties), viewers see that he is not only interested in her. The film begins with Lake's lingering gaze on an older male crossing guard. Later, at the pool where he serves as a lifeguard, Lake rescues an older male swimmer, and runs away when he gets an erection while performing CPR. It is at his next job, at an assisted living facility, where he meets Melvyn Peabody. The film ends with Melvyn's death, after he and Lake have driven across Canada on a sex-filled *Thelma and Louise*-style escapade.

Nude bodies – young and old – are depicted in the film. After Lake tells Melvyn that he 'likes the way you look *now*', we see Melvyn reclining in his bed, nude, and Lake drawing him in his sketch book. The camera – and Lake's eyes – trace down his body, lingering on his flaccid penis. Lake removes his clothing and masturbates. After this scene, Lake's girlfriend Desiree discovers his sketchbook of nude older people and a nurse catches Lake and Melvyn in various stages of undress. He and Desiree break up, and his mother angrily tells him, 'Everyone knows about you and that old man, it's not right … it's disgusting.' Later, Desiree helps Lake bust Melvyn out of the facility. She tells him, 'I think that what you're doing and who you are … it's really brave. And the fact that you're acting on it, it's revolutionary.' As Lake and Melvyn travel across Canada to fulfill Melyvn's wish of seeing the Pacific Ocean again, they sleep in hotels together. Although there are no depictions of sex, viewers do see Lake removing a used condom. There is also a beautiful scene of the two in bed together, with the camera lingering in close-up shots on Melvyn's skin – the attention to his neck, chest, and arms mimic Lake's eyeline in the film. Because the camera is often utilised to show viewers Lake's perspective, depictions of bodies and nudity in the film are done so in a loving and curious way. Unlike films that might utilise older bodies in a comedic or grotesque scene, instead we see older bodies in a new light – one that is appreciative and loving.

Gerontophilia also reverses stereotypes. In two different scenes during Lake and Melvyn's travel across Canada, we see Lake grow jealous when Melvyn chats with younger men. Viewers might expect Melvyn to be the more insecure figure, as he is older than Lake. However, Lake is depicted as the jealous one, perhaps due to his inexperience. In both scenes, Melvyn seems upset with Lake's overreactions – one erupting in violence, as he tosses a birthday cake on one young man who has been chatting with Melvyn. Although no discussion occurs, beside Melvyn's annoyed facial expressions and a surprised retort, 'don't tell me you're jealous!', it is clear that Melvyn is more mature than Lake in multiple ways. Viewers also learn that Melvyn's romantic life has been very complicated, including a marriage to a woman and a son embarrassed of having an 'old queen for a father'. Lake has much to learn from Melvyn and fitting that during Lake's confession that their relationship might be 'more than just sex' for him, Lake discovers that Melvyn has died sometime earlier during the evening. Here, by making Melyvn absent for Lake's confession, the film indicates that their relationship was meant to be one based on sex, and not love. Interestingly, the film ends with Lake returning to and chatting with the elder crossing guard who caught his eye at the beginning of the film. Viewers see that Lake and Melvyn's experiences together served to strengthen Lake's sense of sexual identity while also giving Melvyn a final sexy adventure.

Gerontophilia not only depicts an interracial relationship (Melvyn is black, Lake is white), but also strikes new ground in representing desire, ageing bodies, and more. As Eckert and Martin write,

> By analysing the desire between the protagonists in *Gerontophilia*, Eckert (2017) shows how the camera enables queer images and possibilities through a specific aesthetics that could be described as a queering symmetry between bodies, gazes, contacts, visibilities. By using this queering symmetry as a mode of thinking, the film presents new possibilities of the relationships between ageing, gendering, desiring, and embodying. (2018: par. 28)

In an interview, director Bruce La Bruce discusses the film and his directorial goals. He says,

> But I also think the way that the sexuality of old people is portrayed in pop culture is not romantic in any way. It's presented as something grotesque or ridiculous. Or it's not even acknowledged. To do it in a romantic way and make it believable was part of the strategy of the movie: to show that it can exist and that old people have the same impulses as young people. Sexuality and romance don't just go away. (Martinez, 2015: par. 10)

Not only does the film depict Lake's fetish, but it also depicts a sexual relationship that is not necessarily based on romance – while, as I have discussed, Lake and Melvyn enjoy one another's companionship, the film emphasises Lake's desire for Melyvn, a sexual attraction between younger and older bodies.

Conclusion

Although recent studies illustrate that ageing people have diverse and pleasurable sexual lives, filmic portrayals do not reflect this reality. As baby boomers move into retirement (and into the older person category) there will be a dramatic increase of older people in the population. As well, there will be a corresponding increase in depictions of older people in films and novels. For these portrayals to reflect their potential audiences, they will need to more accurately reflect the dynamic sexual lives of the population. And, as some scholars have noted, diverse representations are also important for individuals to gain knowledge about those who are being represented. The three films analysed in this chapter show how ageing people and sexuality can be portrayed in ways that defy stereotypes and also offer new ways for thinking about what counts as sex and as intimacy. *Cloud 9* portrays nude, ageing people who are both desiring and desirable and also offers alternative forms of intimacy. *Boynton Beach Club* offers multiple representations of widowed older people with very active dating and sexual lives. *Gerontophilia* depicts a queer 'May–December' sexual relationship, emphasising the desirability of older peoples' bodies and upsetting harmful queer stereotypes by playfully reversing them. Tiina Vares (2009: 524) suggests that diverse representations of ageing bodies and sexualities can allow us to 'change our minds about our bodies', that new representations can disrupt historically and culturally specific bodily knowledges, further underscoring the importance and the need for new dynamic and diverse portrayals of ageing people and their sexual lives. More specifically, the three films analysed in this chapter provide diverse representation of the sexual lives of ageing people, yet conversely, are at times limited in the forms of punchlines and reconfigurations of monogamy. Ultimately, all three films portray the resexualisation of older men and women, defying stereotypes of gender and age.

References

Allen, K. and Roberto, K. (2009) From sexism to sexy: challenging young adults' ageism about older women's sexuality, *Sexuality Research & Social Policy*, 6(4): 13–24.

Bouman, W. and Kleinplatz, P. (2015) Moving towards understanding greater diversity and fluidity of sexual expression of older people, *Sexual and Relationship Therapy*, 30: 1–3.

Ebert, R. (2006) Aches on a pain, RogerEbert.com [online], Available from: https://www.rogerebert.com/reviews/boynton-beach-club-2006

Ebert, R. (2009) Be my life's companion, though we'll most certainly grow old, RogerEbert.com [online], Available from: https://www.rogerebert.com/reviews/cloud-nine-2009

Eckert, L. and Martin, S. (2018) Doing age and doing desire in and through film. Queer perspectives on gender, aging, and desire, *Frontiers in Sociology*, 3: 10.

Gatling, M., Mills, J. and Lindsay, D. (2017) Sex after 60? You've got to be joking! Senior sexuality in comedy film, *Journal of Aging Studies*, 40: 23–38.

Gewirtz-Meydan, A., Hafford-Letchfield, T., Ayalon, L., Benyamini, Y., Biermann, V., Coffey, A., Jackson, J., Phelan, A., Voß, P., Zeman, M. and Zeman, Z. (2019) How do older people discuss their own sexuality? A systematic review of qualitative research studies, *Culture, Health & Sexuality*, 21(3): 293–308.

Lauzen, M. and Dozier, D. (2005) Maintaining the double standard: portrayals of age and gender in popular films, *Sex Roles*, 52(7): 437–46.

Malta, S. and Farquharson, K. (2012) The initiation and progression of late-life romantic relationships, *Journal of Sociology*, 50(3): 237–51.

Martinez, R. (2015) Bruce LaBruce on oldies, *Crash Magazine* [online], Available from: https://www.crash.fr/bruce-labruce-interview/

Montemurro, B. and Chewning, L. (2017) Unscripted: exploring representations of older unpartnered women's sexuality, *Journal of Women & Aging*, 30(2): 127–44.

Rowntree, M. (2015) The influence of ageing on baby boomers' not so straight sexualities, *Sexualities*, 18(8): 980–96.

Rubin, J., Moors, A., Matsick, J., Ziegler., A. and Conley, T. (2014) On the margins: considering diversity among consensually non-monogamous relationships, *Journal für Psychologie*, 22(1): 19–37.

Sandberg, L. (2013) Just feeling a naked body close to you: men, sexuality and intimacy in later life, *Sexualities* (3/4): 261–82.

Scherrer, K. (2009) Images of sexuality and aging in gerontological literature, *Sexuality Research & Social Policy*, 6: 5–12.

Sheff, E. (2017) Aging in polyamorous families part two, Psychology Today [online], Available from: https://www.psychologytoday.com/gb/blog/the-polyamorists-next-door/201703/aging-in-polyamorous-families-part-two

Streisand, E. (2016) We're a senior couple who swings with other seniors, Good Housekeeping [online], Available from: https://www.goodhousekeeping.com/life/relationships/a38472/senior-swingers/

Suen, Y-T. (2015) To date or not to date, that is the question: older, single gay men's concerns about dating, *Sexual and Relationship Therapy*, 30: 143–55.

Sun, L. (2019) The representation of later life love in Chinese and European films, *Sexuality & Culture*, 17(3): 203–13.

Vares, T. (2009) Reading the 'sexy oldie': gender, age(ing) and embodiment, *Sexualities*, 12(4): 503–24.

Filmography

Boynton Beach Club (2005) Directed by Susan Seidelmen, Samuel Goldwyn Company.

Cloud 9/Wolke Neun (2008) Directed by Andreas Dresen, Senator Filmverleih.

Gerontophilia (2014) Directed by Bruce La Bruce, Film Option International.

It's Complicated (2009) Directed by Nancy Meyers, Universal Pictures.

4

Resexualisation of older lesbian and gay subjects in film: an analysis of *Cloudburst* and *Gerontophilia*

Paul Simpson and Megan Todd

The idea of later life as a time of fulfilment and diversity is hardly new (see, Gilleard and Higgs, 2000), although such fulfilment is commonly linked to capacity to display perennial youthfulness associated with 'ageing well' or 'successfully'. Curiously, sex and intimacy are rarely mentioned with regard to ageing well (Simpson et al, 2021) and 'ageist erotophobia', the denial of older people as sexual beings, appears endemic (Simpson et al, 2018). Fear, incredulity and disdain for older people's sexuality are entrenched in popular culture, as evident in birthday cards that 'joke' about and equate later life with sexual, physical and cognitive decline (Simpson et al, 2018). Sexuality, intimacy and sexual pleasure remain peripheral to scholarly, policy-related and professional practice literatures on ageing and later life (Simpson et al, 2021). Such concerns indicate a discourse of 'compulsory non-sexuality', which defines older people as 'postsexual' (Simpson, 2021).

Although the misery narrative of a sexless later life is well entrenched, its dominance is by no means complete (Simpson et al, 2021). Accounts of desexualisation or resexualisation as an older lesbian or gay subject are strongly influenced by how ageing sexuality enmeshes with differences of gender, class, race, disability and so on. (See the first edited volume in this book series by Hafford-Letchfield et al, 2021). Unequal opportunities for resexualisation apply both between and within sexual identity categories: one need only contrast esteem and sexual opportunities open to older heterosexual men with those of older lesbian-identified women; and the esteem and opportunities open to older lesbians who differ along lines of class, race and disability (see Harley, 2021; Todd, 2021). As will be seen, however, disadvantaged, older gay and lesbian individuals are by no means lacking capacities to challenge ageism (Simpson, 2015).

Given the relative paucity of literature directly addressing older lesbian and gay people as legitimate sexual agents, we explore the resexualisation of older lesbian and gay subjects through two independently-issued Canadian films. These were chosen from various other films (some of which feature in the next section) because of their more overt sexual references or content, which contribute to the normalisation of older lesbian and gay sexualities. *Cloudburst* (2011) focuses on the longstanding relationship of an old working-class lesbian couple and *Gerontophilia* (2014) focuses on the desire of a young man for an old man and their relationship (see also Chapter 3). We focus on films because they are an engaging method of storytelling and express emotional truths through fiction rather than factual-empirical ones (Plummer, 2001). Films have powerful emotional affects and effects and convey familiar thoughts, feelings, experiences and practices, all of which ground them in reality and help explain social phenomena (see Sutherland and Feltey, 2013). To make sense of the two films, we used a form of thematic analysis that involved two passes through each film by each author: first to note possible themes; and second to produce more in-depth analysis and recalibration of themes. Such a move facilitated agreement on the main themes and their meanings.

Essentially, we show how resexualisation in both films is achieved through thoughts and practice that challenge desexualisation, subvert stereotypes of sexlessness and involve ways of looking (or a particular epistemology), operative in particular, transformative spaces, which enable a 'seeing' of the allure and value of older lesbian and gay sexual subjects.

The 'silvering screen': older people, later life sexuality and older lesbian and gay representation

To contextualise our analysis of *Cloudburst* and *Gerontophilia*, we examine cinematic representations of older people, sexuality in later life and older lesbian and gay characters, featuring mainly in Hollywood and British films since the 1950s, and which index the enmeshments of age with sexuality and gender especially. Exploring key representations affords insight into the uneven fortunes of older lesbian and gay people in the 'reel' and 'real' worlds. Using several literature search databases designed to access scholarship across social sciences, arts and humanities,[1] we found much work devoted to representations of older people and to younger/ageless lesbian and gay characters but much less to older people or older lesbian and gay characters as (valid) sexual beings.

Older people on film

The dominant and enduring motif of the 'silvering screen' (Chivers, 2011) concerns old age as pitiful loss and degeneration of youthful attractiveness, health, self-control and sexuality. This depiction appears in the shape of protagonist, Norma Desmond, in the classic, *Sunset Boulevard* (1950), who represents fallen status, social redundancy, diminution of ability and bodily decay/ageing. Of course, when looked at beyond an all-too-familiar, commonsense narrative of personal failure (of an older female, ex-star now painfully diminished), such a portrayal tells us more about the workings of gender, power, status, stigma and wider societal anxieties about growing old(er) (Chivers, 2011; Dolan, 2018). Such thinking is indicative of a clutch of ageist discourses that perpetuates stereotypes, myths and misconceptions about later life, itself metonymic with the end of sex and sexual identity (Bouman et al, 2006; Simpson, 2021). Besides, older characters are often synonymous with illness and death, social and actual (Sola-Morales, 2020). Such representations of later life are also highly gendered given that, when old(er) female characters in film are not represented as appendages to the lives of (younger) others or families, figuring as (grand-)maternal and supportive (and thus unsexy), they can be constructed as pathological. However, if unattached and independent, they can be seen as a predatory sexual threat, to heteronormative marriage, for example, as a 'cougar' (see Markson, 2003).

Further, a limited range of stereotypes has been observed in relation to older characters. Some characters have been cast nostalgically as emotionally aware if sometimes hidden by a cantankerous front (though physically frail) like the grandfather played by Henry Fonda in *On Golden Pond* (1981). The characters played by John Wayne could be thought to represent a patriotic and stoic later life and in the face of life-ending illness in his last film, *The Shootist* (1976). Later life can also be valorised on film (as in everyday life) when it is seen to mimic an age-defying, youthful vitality. A prime example of the latter is *Cocoon* (1985), which reinforces the notion of ageing/old age as valid when 'youthful' and thus to be endlessly deferred or overcome. Such portrayals can be contrasted with bad-tempered, comedic characters, as in *Grumpy Old Men* (1993) behaving 'badly' and against stereotype and the peevish, passive-aggressive (female-coded), prying, neighbour (Gatling et al, 2017). One example of the latter is Judy Dench's destructive character in *Notes on a Scandal* (2006), though this film does upend the sweet little old lady stereotype. Themes of dependency and isolation also loom large where older people are infantilised or else are subject to cruelty and abuse as in *Nebraska* (2013) and in more extreme form in the psycho-horror (and camp classic), *Whatever Happened to Baby Jane* (1962), which also conflates age with disability and poor mental health, if not derangement.

Nevertheless, there are signs of some critical space within film-making (and British television) where more empowering portrayals of later life/old age are possible but these tend to be exceptional, as well as white and affluent when they do occur (Liddy, 2014). Judy Dench's powerful, octogenarian, 'M', in the Bond-movie *Skyfall* (2012) indexes a rare subversion of conventional representations of old femininity (Eckert and Martin, 2018). Similarly, the British television series, *Last Tango in Halifax* (2012–20), offered a wry look at complex intergenerational intimacies centred on a seventysomething, heterosexual couple.

Later life sexuality on film

In terms of later life sexuality, arguably, the dominant representational motif concerns sexlessness or 'compulsory non-sexuality' (Simpson et al, 2021). Indeed, Gatling et al (2017) have observed how, in the entertainment media, later life itself and ageing sexuality are often framed as comedic, not as something to laugh along with but the butt of humour and ridicule, which indicates the workings of ageist erotophobia (Simpson, 2021). Besides, later life sexuality often seems freighted with drama, as visible in *The Best Exotic Marigold Hotel* (2011), which homogenises older characters aged between their fifties and seventies. Later life sexuality has also been portrayed as fraught with anxiety, as in *Hope Springs* (2012), where an older heterosexual couple struggles in communicating sexual needs. While the two latter films at least recognise the existence of sex in later life, they reinforce the notion that ageing sexuality is 'unwatchable' (Walz, 2002) and thus unworthy of association with legitimate desire. Sex in later life can be talked about as a problem but not seen as a pleasurable experience.

There have been some notable attempts to challenge later life asexual stereotypes, as represented in the 'May–December' relationship of *Harold and Maude* (1971), though, to make it palatable, the film was marketed as a 'black comedy'. The father-son road movie, *Nebraska* (2013) also portrays various older characters as sexual subjects. Although involving an interesting reversal of discourse, and despite attempts to foreground, diversify and sexualise older characters and legitimise intergenerational intimacy, such representations remain largely heteronormative (Chivers, 2011). Nevertheless, Gatling et al (2017) note that *Beginners* (2010) represents a welcome exception to the norm, which involves a seventysomething man (played by Hollywood icon, Christopher Plummer), who 'comes out' after his wife's death and whose non-monogamous gay lifestyle is normalised.

Older lesbian and gay sexualities on film

To understand representations of non-normative ageing sexualities on film, we need to consider a brief, complex history of representations of lesbian and gay characters generally over the past 70 years or so. A cursory review of film studies literature soon reveals that lesbian and gay cinematic representation, despite more recent gains in 'tolerance', continues to be marked by various forms of pathology. Lesbian and gay characters have been persistently caricatured as gender deviants, sexual inverts and perverts (Tran, 2019), as apparent in the effeminate 'sissy', the predator, the mannish woman or, more exotically, the lesbian vampire (Russo, 1976/1987). Essentially, lesbian and gay characters have been subjected to a range of restricted portrayals from more or less invisibility to that of villain or victim and one worthy of punishment, as quite recently suggested in *Disobedience* (2017) where a lesbian relationship is portrayed as illicit and thus doomed. It has also been observed that even more liberal interpretations of sexual difference have reinforced heteronormative thinking (Dyer, 1978; Tran, 2019). However, we refer later to some complex and more positively-coded representations.

When considering older lesbian and gay characters on film, of particular significance is representation of the self-torturing (a common trope) and/or sadistic queer figure (Russo, 1976/1987), which is evident in the film of an early 1960s play, *The Killing of Sister George* (1968). Here, the older lesbian protagonist, June Buckridge/Sister George, is represented as a grotesque who abuses her younger, femme lover, 'Childie'. Their sexual relationship is amply suggested in a scene where they rehearse as Laurel and Hardy for a fancy dress party, though in a way that indicates sadistic control and exploitation by the older woman. If *Victim* (1961) (based on extortion of a younger gay man) ends in the self-annihilation of a central character, (via suicide to escape stigma), *Sister George* culminates in the symbolic annihilation of June as a person and George as a television soap star. June's/George's downfall, attributable to *public* display of her sexuality, is facilitated by her nemesis, the ironically named television producer, 'Miss Mercy', whose middle-aged, manicured femininity conceals a steely, ruthless (masculine-coded but closeted) calculation that expropriates June/George of livelihood and lover. In contrast, a queer re-reading of *George* would argue that June represents a disruptive, angry, carnivalesque, sexualised version of older lesbian identity[2] that is redolent of the sweary, butch, old dyke in *Cloudburst*.

However, the tolerance dividend that has developed in Britain, the US and parts of Europe over the past 25 years or so has seen the emergence of representations that could be described as 'post-queer' with more 'mainstream' appeal where stigma, pathology and angry, oppositional politics are no longer represented as central or necessary to lesbian and gay identity and experience. The category just described could include *Beginners* (2010), which involves the protagonist in an open relationship with a younger man. In contrast, the biopic, *Behind the Candelabra*, based on celebrity pianist-showman, Liberace (2013), reminds us that not all queer later life self-sexualisation is egalitarian and life-affirming. This film is significant for depicting how an older, narcissistic gay celebrity (re)sexualises himself at the cost of his younger and later spurned lover.

There are also several independent films in the same category (and beyond Hollywood), featuring older lesbians as central characters that mix comedy with the normalisation of difference and create a critical, cultural-political space. *So, My Grandma's a Lesbian!/Salir del Ropero* (Spanish title: 'Coming out of the Closet') (2019) mixes strong and vulnerable female characters, intergenerational political conflict, subversion of authority figures (a priest) and slapstick and observational comedy with feel-good factor. *Sand Dollars* (2014) depicts a French woman, Anne (Geraldine Chaplin), in her seventies, who pays for the company and body of a much younger, Dominican woman, Noeli, in her early twenties. This film subverts stereotypes of the sexless older woman and the male-oriented sex tourist narrative. In *Tru Love* (2013), Alice, a recent widow in her early sixties, visits her workaholic daughter and ends up in a relationship with her daughter's friend, thirtysomething, Tru. Here, Alice is represented as both desirable, (several younger lesbians eye her up), and empowered to act upon long-repressed desires. This category could easily accommodate the two films selected for in-depth analysis, which offer refreshing challenges to the stereotypical representations described earlier.

Analysis: *Cloudburst* and *Gerontophilia*

The stories in outline

Cloudburst stars Olympia Dukakis as 'Stella' and Brenda Fricker as 'Dotty', who are co-habiting lovers of 31 years. Dotty has an age-related visual impairment and is practically cared for by Stella. Their lesbian (and class) status is quickly established by masculine, truck-driving Stella, listening to k. d. lang, returning to their cat-filled, chaotically presented home in Maine, US. The couple is not 'out' to Dotty's staid, homo/lesbophobic granddaughter who is oblivious to their relationship. Effectively, the plot begins when Dotty is tricked by her granddaughter into being taken into institutional care and thus placed beyond what Molly sees as Stella's malign influence. However, Dotty is liberated by Stella and they go on the road to escape over the border into Canada (road movies being more often associated with youth and development rather than age/maturity fixed into place) where they can legally marry and thus remain inseparable. Along the way, they pick up a handsome young male Canadian hitch-hiker and (self-proclaimed) 'modern dance' practitioner, Prentice. After several skirmishes with the law and Prentice's redneck stepfather, they become friends until Dotty's sudden death. Like *Gerontophilia*, *Cloudburst* uses humour to address serious issues, including elder abuse, stigmatised identity and the interlocking constraints of being a working-class, disabled, older lesbian. Kehoe's (1986) phrase 'triply invisible' resonates here, as the film draws attention to the multiple oppressions that can constrain older lesbian lives. Despite such constraints, the couple manages to escape one-dimensional victimhood and asserts the value of their relationship.

Although with a less well-recognised cast, *Gerontophilia* is directed by queer filmmaker, Bruce LaBruce. It tells a story of intersectional disadvantage, (concerning age and sexual differences), through 18-year-old, bisexual,

Lake's desire for old men and especially through his developing love for 80-year-old, gay-identified, astute, sardonic, biracial Melvyn, who he meets when working in a care home for older people. Increasingly appalled at the ageism rife within the 'care' home's regime that controls residents through medication and the home's punitive reaction to the intimacy/relationship developing between himself and Melvyn, using his mother's car, Lake liberates Melvyn from the care home and they set off on the road from Quebec (East Coast) to the Canadian Pacific Coast. The journey is motivated by Melvyn's longing to see the West Coast again (possibly for the last time) and suggests use not just of subversive content/themes but also of 'the road' as associated with contingency, fluidity, mobility and agency. En route, the protagonists experience various adventures and fall in love until Melvyn's sudden death, which helps reconcile Lake with his mother, Marie, his ex-girlfriend, Desirée, and Melvyn's estranged (middle-aged) son and, crucially, Lake with his own sexual desires for old men.

Older bodies that matter: challenging desexualisation

Despite Dotty's frailties and visual impairment, *Cloudburst* avoids pathologising her ageing, classed and disabled body. Her body may fall short of the youthful ideal (Twigg, 2013) and she is referred to affectionately as a 'Teletubby', a 'cow' and 'fat'. She is presented as caring and in need of physical care but the restrictive and harmful framing of old age as decline is presented here as the product of ageist attitudes. Dotty's age-related visual impairment is conceptualised as strength: while she does not 'see'; she has enhanced understanding (which avoids disablism in decoupling sight from knowledge/understanding). She is also well aware of Stella's fears stemming from living as a lesbian during a sexually conservative era, and her squeamishness about the male anatomy, despite her potty mouth, remarking to Prentice that Stella would 'faint if she saw your balls'. In effect, the older women's ageing, classed sexuality is presented as a form of power which has the potential to challenge and shift dominant constructions of power. In effect, the film plays with sexist and ageist expectations about women's appearance and behaviours. Far from being 'unwatchable' in later life (Woodward, 1991: Walz, 2002), the women's embodied selves demand and capture our attention and that we 'see' them, and Stella in particular, as active, independent and powerful (Gill, 2008). Here, we see a depiction of older, working-class women/lesbians, which transcends both the begrudged 'sexy oldie' and 'asexual old age' stereotypes, and challenges heteronormative assumptions of ageing.

Interestingly, while most references to sex and intimacy occur between Stella and Dotty, we only see men naked in this film (Prentice and his stepfather). On all occasions, the potency of the male body is challenged in comedic ways. Also, it is Dotty who is, on one occasion, literally, faced with a penis. Even the dildo (in an early scene), as phallic replacement, serves as a source of humour. The film suggests a resistance to conventional understandings of the operation of power. It reverses power relations so that power is less associated with youthful heteropatriarchal masculinity than with mature/old(er) lesbian femininity. We could, then, ask: Why does the film not depict sex and older lesbian bodies more overtly? Could this be a deliberate choice to avoid potential appropriation/titillation by male heterosexual audiences? Or, would depiction of so-called abject bodies be too subversive even for a lesbian audience? We argue that it matters less whether we are given an actual depiction of sex and desire in (lesbian) old age. What is more important is the way the film constructs older working-class lesbian desire as everyday and how it also creates connections between past, present and future desires. We can sense how the embodied desire and passion between Dotty and Stella has developed through the years. Desire between the women is still present in their relationship through humour and their declarations and memories. One scene, which informs the film's title, has a sudden cloudburst that prompts Stella and Dotty to leave their truck to enjoy the sensation of the rain, from which ensues a long, passionate kiss suggestive of years of love, desire and now liberation.

Gerontophilia also shows that ageing (gay male) bodies matter, though, in radically different and at times in highly ambivalent ways. Lake's attraction to older male bodies is established early in the film where he is seen (in slow-motion) looking longingly at an old, male street-crossing attendant. His gay gerontophilic desire is also suggested in the quality of his drawing of an old man swimming while working as a pool lifeguard. While drawing the older swimmer, Lake suddenly notices him lying face-down floating in the pool and dives into to rescue him. After giving mouth-to-mouth resuscitation, we see that two teenaged female onlookers notice less that Lake has acted ethically in trying to save a life than that he appears to have ejaculated or may at least have developed an erection. The incident, while ambiguous, is shown as occasion for acute shame, as represented in Lake's hasty withdrawal from the scene, hand hiding his groin and his subsequent sacking.

Subverting sexless stereotypes: escaping the constructions of old age

Another theme evident in both films concerns the dismantling of stereotypes and ludic reassertion of ageing sexuality. Unlike films featured in our earlier review, humour figures differently and we are invited to laugh with and not at the protagonists. *Cloudburst* quickly establishes an easy sexual intimacy between the two women. For example, Dotty asks Stella what it means 'to Swiffer' (a reference to a mop), joking that the women on the TV adverts talk about it like something which can give multiple orgasms. An early scene involves Stella, watching a lesbian porn film which Dotty tells her is made for heterosexual men. Stella's response and enjoyment regardless of this, serves as a 'troubling' of the 'male gaze' (Mulvey, 1975) and reappropriation of pornography that is about but not made for lesbian-identified women. When Dotty is being bundled out of their shared home, Stella subverts age and sexuality when she shouts at her son-in-law policeman, 'I am not your grandma … but I did get to second base with her in the seventh grade'. When on the road, Stella declares to Prentice 'If I were on death row, I'd request my final meal be right between k.d. lang's legs'. Perhaps most startling of all, once transformed from the headscarf-wearing grandmother figure she fakes to hitch a lift to Canada, she shocks her prurient, middle-aged male driver, with her eulogy on the value of an accommodating 'cunt', which further challenges stereotypes about appropriate older female taste and comportment. Simultaneously, Stella's eulogy challenges the driver's sexist, phallocentric, ageist and heteronormative valuing of a 'snug' (youthful) 'vagina', itself a medical term that Stella likens to 'a disease'.

While tempting to see Dotty as the familiar, frail, sweet old lady, helpless and naïve, and 'the femme partner', she confounds expectations and sexual norms when she casually intones: 'Imagine: you can now buy lesbian porn at the gas station' and, when considering the (heteronormative) marriage license form later in the film, asks which of them should be named on it as the 'bachelor'. A comic interlude with a dildo (the ownership of a sex toy further troubles the myth of lesbian bed-death, though it isn't used in quite the way it is intended!), ends up with Dotty falling out of bed, hurting herself and, when recuperating in hospital, she tells Stella that it will be 'six weeks before you can slap my arse again'. The contrast between who Stella and Dotty actually 'are' and their performances, reveal the ways in which many of the problems of ageing are linked to ageism rather than old age itself. In *Cloudburst*, older lesbian sexuality is not made invisible, as the camera lingers on the protagonists' faces, again, challenging the idea of the 'unwatchability' of old age/femininity (Woodward, 1991) and the taboo of later life sexuality.

Similarly, a comedic section in *Gerontophilia* sees Lake and Melvyn in their underwear (suggesting erotic and bodily equality), getting drunk and playing cards (see also later). Although the narrative is seen largely through the younger character, Melvyn is not simply resexualised by the younger party. He is too savvy and emotionally independent to require motivation or approval by others but his relationship with Lake does offer a new lease of life towards the end of his life and seems to make sex more vital at this point in the life course (see Rennie, 2021). It is arguable that Melvyn's desiring and being desired by Lake indicates, like Dotty and Stella, the operation of an alternative, mutual, egalitarian relationship that undercuts or queers common expectations of ageing, gendered, (classed and raced) sexuality.

Moreover, the carcereal treatment of residents in care homes prompts Stella and Lake respectively to take action to liberate their lovers. While both are determined, their mood and strategies are, again, radically different. To free Dotty from the care home, Stella transforms into an aged stereotype with a headscarf, nightdress and walking stick (a 'dragging-up'-cum-'ageing-up'). When passing as old, it appears that a straight or gay identity becomes irrelevant under the institutional gaze that renders older people sexless. Thus, Stella becomes invisible to the nurse on duty as anything other than just another, if 'naughty', resident who has been out later than she should.

In contrast, Lake's liberation strategy involves using his mother's car and, justifying his radical action, he reverses the usual discourse in concluding that disgust lies not in older bodies and older people's sexuality, but, rather, in response to their (sexual) relationship, which they feel obliged to hide. In his critical questioning, Lake contrasts his relationship with Melvyn with the control of residents through oppressive attitudes and regimes, involving soporific, mood-altering medication. In a later reconciliation scene, Lake's ex-girlfriend, would-be socialist-feminist revolutionary, Desirée, acknowledges the significance of Lake's transgressive desire for older body-selves as 'truly revolutionary'. Although ambivalent about what she, candidly calls 'the fucked-up part' of Lake's sexual desire, Desirée acknowledges that his attraction to old men 'goes against … expectations of ageing, beauty and what is desirable' thus suggesting the socially-constructed character of such qualities and what we regard as human nature.

Typical of road movies (for example, *Thelma and Louise*, 1991), both films have much to say about liberation from the constraints of conventionality and institutions (that can help construct old age as sexless) as a means of self-reclamation and autonomy. The freedom of the open road references the start of escape from *ageist* oppression (which includes desexualisation and pathologisation), transformation of character and circumstance and the development of close, mutual understanding between the differently-aged protagonists. Following the challenges encountered *en route*, in *Gerontophilia*, Lake's confidence in his desire for old men appears enhanced if beyond stigma and apology (at least for himself) by the end of the film. Following their escape from the home, which controls and oppresses its residents through soporific medication, regimentation and open, ageist contempt among care staff, Melvyn, (like Dotty in *Cloudburst*), is recuperated from a living death of enforced decrepitude and desexualised status.

The optics of allure: older lesbian and gay bodies (in transformative spaces)

Having been dismissed from his job as a pool attendant for getting sexually excited over an old man, Lake secures a job as a care worker in a nursing home that contains old people in the sense of both warehousing and incarcerating them. The disgust at and contempt for old people, who count as beyond the erotic imaginary if not outside of viable life itself, appear institutionalised in the attitudes and everyday practices of staff and care home structures. In particular, we witness the neglect of one male resident wandering aimlessly in a corridor whose hospital gown is open, exposing his naked buttocks. This scene is suggestive of ugliness, a negative aesthetic where age equates with decrepitude, representing the opposite of sexual attractiveness, desirability and value. It is, though, tempting to view, within these perspectival shots (which place the viewer in Lake's shoes), the ageist contempt that suffuses the care home, as pivotal in transforming Lake's thinking into more critical and subversive mode. This is suggested when we glimpse, in slow-motion through Lake's erotic gaze, resignification of the older male resident's buttocks as desirable.

In several scenes, Lake's drawings of older men appear to re-aestheticise the marks of ageing (see also Chapter 2), suggesting erotic appreciation of older male bodies as worthy of the artistic and erotic gaze. Lake's desire for and valuing of the old male body is particularly evident when he draws a picture of a sleeping Melvyn and pulls back the bedclothes to view the latter's naked body while he masturbates into his own trousers. At several points in the film and during their love-making, it is significant that the camera lingers over Melvyn's rather than Lake's body, suggesting, against conventional expectations, (re)aestheticisation of the older body as the focus of desire.

The scenes just described are indicative of a reversal of the usual aesthetic of youth as the standard of beauty and attractiveness. Significantly, it is Lake who appears throughout the film as the viewing and desiring subject given that the camera more often shows us what he is seeing and at times lingers over Melvyn's body as the *subject* of desire. This contrasts with films like *Death in Venice* (1971) that instantiate the more common focus by the older man on the younger man as the *object* of desire. Not only does this reversal resignify older body-selves as worthy of the sexual/erotic gaze, it also indicates possibilities for the inclusion of older gay men (and older people more generally) within the sexual imaginary. This re-signification is particularly important given the prevalence of accounts of 'accelerated ageing' in gay male cultures where men are commonly viewed as old(er) (and thus subjected to socio-sexual exclusion), well before their heterosexual male peers might expect comparable treatment (Simpson, 2015).

Moreover, in *Cloudburst*, older lesbian body-selves are revalued in two institutional spaces, namely, the home/marriage and the care home, both of which are transcended by being on the road, though the space of freedom represented by the road also prompts transformation in the two main protagonists (as well as Prentice). Freed from these homogenising, invisibilising spaces, the women – often visually thrown into relief against the landscape – become visible and compelling. Like Lake and Melvyn in *Gerontophilia*, Stella, Dotty (and Prentice) are searching for a safe space for expression of their embodied sexualities, forcing a negotiation with self-identity and family. Here, the matter is less concerned with families of choice (Weeks et al, 2001), though Stella and Dotty become a more interesting, rootless, surrogate family with Prentice, but connected to communities of understanding able to hear one's joys, suffering and situation (Plummer, 1995). References to lesbian culture are made throughout, from k. d. lang to Ellen and Portia, Rosie O'Donnell and 'Jesus Anne Heche Christ', and a soundtrack filled with lesbian singer/songwriters. The film also addresses a range of boundaries and borders, those between youth and age, land and sea, Canada and the US and bodily borders too such as Prentice's cavity search when crossing into Canada! In their treatment, such borders are shown largely as fluid, permeable and mutable (and darkly comedic in the latter case).

Finally, the Canadian open road and seascape in *Cloudburst* offer not just a beautiful backdrop but are also spaces that offer the possibility of transformation and practically become characters in their own right. The road movie narrative in both films evokes the familiar tropes of rebellion, freedom, and the outlaw couple (again, think *Thelma and Louise*), frequently associated with such films (Laderman, 1996). The road can also be seen as a metaphor for the life course and, along with the sea and the film itself, becomes a space and symbol of liberation from reductive social expectations of ageing, gendered sexual difference.

Concluding thoughts

Cloudburst and *Gerontophilia* help illuminate the complex workings of power concerning valid sexual citizenship along intersectional lines of age, sexuality, class (and race in the case of the latter). Both stories offer a vision of resexualisation possible through forms of representation, namely, thought and practice that: question desexualisation; subvert stereotypes of sexlessness to help enact an older sexual self; and offer critical ways of looking in spaces that make visible the allure and value of older lesbian and gay sexual subjectivities.

Themes explored in the films reference other important cultural-political issues. In their several ways, Stella, Dotty and Melvyn transcend and show us something more complicated than the dominant, polar paradigms of ageing as irrecoverable decline and isolation or as 'successful' (Gullette, 2004). In contrast to films like *The Kids Are Alright* (2010), accused of erasing feminist and queer critiques of sexual and gender normativity (Walters, 2012), *Cloudburst* celebrates lesbian desire and culture while *Gerontophilia* celebrates gay cross-generational conviviality and desire, both often considered lacking in gay male cultures (Simpson, 2015). Although there might not be a lesbian community around Stella and Dotty, perhaps not surprising given their age and Stella's past heterosexual experiences, nor any gay kinship supporting

Lake and Melvyn, there is, in both films, a celebration of the age-inflected forms of sexual difference and relatedness that they embody.

Despite the lack of a wider network able to hear the protagonists' stories, in *Cloudburst* there are clear lesbian-feminist re-imaginings of ageing intimacy and inclusive kinship that involve critique of conventional family. Dotty compares her experience of heterosexual marriage to a brain clot, describing it as 'a crock of shite for helpless men and confused women' and something for 'normal' people. In *Gerontophilia*, heterosexual marriage and conventional family had been felt as a generational obligation for Melvyn who spoke of them in terms of alienation and rejection. His son was described as 'embarrassed by an old queen for a father' and had not introduced Melvyn to his own grandson. In contrast to his relationship with Lake, Melvyn speaks of rejection by biological family because of his sexuality and fellow gay men because of his age thus invoking the double jeopardy faced by older lesbian and gay people who experience exclusion on the grounds of sexuality combined with age/desirability (Simpson et al, 2018). Yet, poignantly, after Melvyn's funeral, (itself a reconciliation scene), and at the point of Dotty's death, we glimpse the more supportive, though intriguingly 'dysfunctional', families that could have been.

Further, both films suggest a queering of ageing sexuality and more than a nod to the 'new gay/lesbian sincerity' in films as identified by Moor (2018), which mixes cultural politics with claims to the authenticity and viability of queer lives. Each film challenges entrenched stereotypes concerning the emotional and sexual aridity of long-term lesbian relationships ('bed-death') and the impossibility of cross-generational ('May–December') relationships as unnatural or taboo (Richardson, 2020). All the old characters (in their seventies and eighties) remain legitimate sexual citizens (Richardson, 2017) and in ways that avoid fetishisation of old age. In effect, the films present the main characters' relationships as valid and can be contrasted with the more dishonest, if flaky, superficial, heterosexual relations spoken of by Prentice in *Cloudburst* and practiced by Lake's mother, Marie, in *Gerontophilia*. The depictions in both films also offer an alternative aesthetics whereby older bodies are understood as sexually desirable, worthy of the erotic gaze and are thus rescued from ugliness, decrepitude and stigma. Such negative qualities seem unthinkable in relation to *Cloudburst* but this recuperative project ramifies especially in *Gerontophilia* given the more intense ageism characteristic of 'Western' gay male cultures (Simpson, 2015).

Finally, not only do both films offer strategies and resources to challenge compulsory non-sexuality and ageist erotophobia (Simpson, 2021) as applied to older lesbian and gay people, but also their reversals of discourse challenge the assumed stable ontology of categories of age, sexuality (and ageing sexuality) and thus who is allowed to desire whom. Such considerations are hugely important as they dovetail with issues of erotic equality and democracy as well as quality of life in old age.

Notes

1 Proquest/Applied Social Sciences Index and Abstracts (ASSIA), Scopus and Google Scholar.

2 Sincere thanks to Dr Andrew Moor, former Reader in Cinematic History, Manchester Metropolitan University, for his invaluable insights and commentary.

References

Bouman, W.P., Arcelus, J. and Benbow, S.M. (2006) Nottingham Study of Sexuality and Ageing (NoSSA I). Attitudes regarding sexuality and older people: a review of the literature, *Sexual and Relationship Therapy*, 21(2): 149–61.

Chivers, S. (2011) *The Silvering Screen: Old Age and Disability in Cinema*, University of Toronto Press.

Dolan, J. (2018) *Contemporary Cinema and 'Old Age': Gender and the Silvering of Stardom*, Palgrave Macmillan.

Dyer, R. (1978) Gays in film, *Jump Cut: A Review of Contemporary Media*, 18(1): 5–16.

Eckert, L. and Martin, S. (2018) Doing age and doing desire in and through film: queer perspectives on gender, aging, and desire, *Frontiers in Sociology*, 3: 10.

Gatling, M., Mills, J. and Lindsay, D. (2017) Sex after 60? You've got to be joking: senior sexuality in comedy film, *Journal of Aging Studies*, 40(1): 23–8.

Gill, R. (2008). Empowerment/sexism: figuring female sexual agency in contemporary advertising, *Feminism and Psychology*, 18(1): 35–60.

Gilleard, C. and Higgs, P. (2000) *Cultures of Ageing: Self, Citizen and the Body*, Pearson Educational Limited.

Gullette, M. (2004) *Aged by Culture*, The University of Chicago Press.

Hafford-Letchfield, T., Simpson, P. and Reynolds, P. (eds) (2021) *Sex and Diversity in Later Life: Critical Perspectives*, Bristol: Policy Press.

Harley, D. (2021) Sexual expression and pleasure among black minority ethnic older women, in T. Hafford-Letchfield, P. Simpson and P. Reynolds (eds) (2021) *Sex and Diversity in Later Life: Critical Perspectives*, Policy Press, pp 15–37.

Kehoe, M. (1986) Lesbians over sixty-five: a triply invisible minority, *Journal of Homosexuality*, 12(3–4): 139–52.

Laderman, D. (2002) *Driving Visions: Exploring the Road Movie*, University of Texas Press.

Liddy, S. (2014) 'Missing persons'? Representations of mature female sexuality in British and Irish Film 1998–2011, *Postgraduate Journal of Women, Ageing and Media*, 1: 33–58.

Markson, E. (2003) The female aging body through film, in C. Faircloth (ed) *Aging Bodies, Images and Everyday Experiences*, Alta Mira Press, pp 77–102.
Moor, A. (2018) 'New gay sincerity' and Andrew Haigh's *Weekend* (UK, 2011), *Film Studies*, 19(1): 4–19.
Mulvey, L. (1975) Visual pleasure and narrative cinema, *Screen*, 16(3): 6–18.
Plummer, K. (1995) *Telling Sexual Stories: Power, Change and Social Worlds*, Routledge.
Plummer, K. (2001) *Documents of Life 2: An Invitation to a Critical Humanism*, Sage Publications.
Rennie, K. (2021) Sexual desires and intimacy needs in older persons and towards the end of life, in T. Hafford-Letchfield, P. Simpson and P. Reynolds (eds) *Sex and Diversity in Later Life: Critical Perspectives*, Policy Press, 39–55.
Richardson, D. (2017) Rethinking sexual citizenship, *Sociology*, 51(2): 208–24.
Richardson, N. (2020) Ageing predators and asexual old queens: challenging stereotypes of cross-generational gay relationships in *Beginners* and *Gerontophilia*, in J. Gwynne and N. Richardson (eds) *Cross-Generational Relationships and Cinema*, Palgrave Macmillan, pp 105–22.
Russo, V. (1976/1987) *The Celluloid Closet: Homosexuality in the Movies*, Harper Row.
Simpson, P. (2015) *Middle-aged Gay Men, Ageing and Ageism: Over the Rainbow?* Palgrave Macmillan.
Simpson, P. (2021) At your age???!!! The constraints of ageist erotophobia on older people's sexual and intimate relationships, in P. Simpson, P. Reynolds and T. Hafford-Letchfield (eds) *Desexualisation in Later Life: The Limits of Sex and Intimacy*, Policy Press, pp 35–51.
Simpson, P., Reynolds, P. and Hafford-Letchfield, T. (eds) (2021) *Desexualisation in Later Life: the Limits of Sex and Intimacy*, Policy Press.
Simpson, P., Wilson, C., Brown, L.J.E., Dickinson, T. and Horne, M. (2018) 'We've had our sex life way back': older care home residents, sexuality and intimacy, *Ageing & Society*, 38(7): 1478–501.
Sola-Morales, S. (2020) Older people, grandparents: how men age in the cinema, in J. Rey (ed) *Men on the Screen: Re-visions of Masculinity in Spanish Cinema 1939–2019*, Peter Lang, 237–47.
Sutherland, J.-A. and Feltey, C. (eds) (2013) *Cinematic Sociology: Social Life in Film* (2nd edn), Sage.
Todd, M. (2021) Thinking the unthinkable: older lesbians, sex and violence, in T. Hafford-Letchfield, P. Simpson and P. Reynolds (eds) *Sex and Diversity in Later Life: Critical Perspectives*, Policy Press, 121–38.
Tran, L. (2019) Queer history through a Hollywood lens, *Augsburg Honors Review*, 12(9): 130–9.
Twigg, J. (2013) *Fashion and Age: Dress, the Body and Later Life*, A&C Black.
Walters, S.D. (2012) The kids are all right but the lesbians aren't: queer kinship in US culture, *Sexualities*, 15(8): 917–33.

Walz, T. (2002) Crones, dirty old men, sexy seniors: representations of the sexuality of older persons, *Journal of Aging and Identity*, 7(2): 99–112.

Weeks, J., Heaphy, B. and Donovan, C. (2001) *Same Sex Intimacies: Families of Choice and Other Life Experiments*, Routledge.

Woodward, K. (1991) *Ageing and its Discontents: Freud and Other Fictions*, Indiana University Press.

Filmography

Beginners (2010) Mike Mills, US: Focus Features.

Behind the Candelabra (2013) Steven Soderbergh, US: HBO Films.

Cloudburst (2011) Thom Fitzgerald, Canada: Sidney Kimmel Entertainment.

Cocoon (1985) Ron Howard, US: 20th Century Fox.

Death in Venice (1971) Lucino Visconti, Italy/France: Warner Bros.

Disobedience (2017) Sebastian Lelio, UK: Curzon Artificial Eye.

Gerontophilia (2014) Bruce LaBruce, Canada: Film Option International.

Grumpy Old Men (1993) Donald Petrie, US: Warner Bros.

Harold and Maude (1971) Hal Ashby, US: Paramount Pictures.

Hope Springs (2012) David Frankel, US: Sony Pictures Releasing/Lionsgate.

Last Tango in Halifax (2012–2020) (Various directors) Sally Wainwright, UK: BBC1.

Nebraska (2013) Alexander Payne, UK/US: Paramount Vantage.

Notes on a Scandal (2006) Richard Eyre, UK: Fox Searchlight Pictures.

On Golden Pond (1981) Mark Rydell, US: Universal Pictures.

The Best Exotic Marigold Hotel (2011) John Madden, UK: Fox Searchlight Pictures.

The Kids Are All Right (2010) Lisa Cholodenko, US: Focus Features.

The Killing of Sister George (1968) Robert Aldrich, US: Cinerama Releasing Corporation.

The Shootist (1976) Don Segal, US: Paramount Pictures/Dino de Laurentis Company (International).

Sand Dollars (2014) Israel Cárdenas and Laura Amelia Guzmán, Spain: FiGa.

Skyfall (2012) Sam Mendes, London: Eon Productions.

So, My Grandma's A Lesbian!/Salir del Ropero (2019) Ángeles Reiné, Spain: Netflix.

Sunset Boulevard (1950) Billy Wilder, US: Paramount Pictures.

Thelma and Louise (1991) Ridley Scott, US: Metro-Goldwyn-Mayer.

Tru Love (2013) Kate Johnston and Shauna MacDonald, Canada: IndieCan Entertainment/Wolfe Releasing.

Victim (1961) Basil Dearden, UK: Rank Film Distributors.

Whatever Happened to Baby Jane (1962) Robert Aldrich, US: Warner Bros. Pictures.

5

Resexualisation, later life and kink

Paul Reynolds

Much of the discussion of sex and intimacy in later life builds on two desexualising elements: the physiological and the aesthetic. The physiological focuses on sexual function/dysfunction (tied to the strong connection of sex as essentially penetrative, genito-centric and traditionally associated with fertility and reproduction) and the impact of different health conditions on sexual appetite and function. These impacts include: erectile dysfunction and pain and discomfort arising from less vaginal lubrication and menopause; bodily change (ageing and infirmity) that departs from stereotypical notions of beauty and attraction, producing diminished desire; and changes interpreted as difficulties in achieving orgasm (it might take longer or happen less). These developments are interpreted within a context where the 'natural' sexual life course model starts as a teenager with puberty and finishes into the third age (50+). It is borne of the performative construction of sex as a practice characterised by rampant desire, athleticism, virility and fertility, combined with a life cycle that detaches sex from dignity and 'appropriateness' as people age.

This is the conceptual basis by which older people suffer an ageist erotophobia, which constitutes an active desexualisation rather than a 'natural' or 'normal' process as it is represented on a surface level (Simpson, 2015). The 'normal' life course model offers inexorable sexual diminishment as the body ages. This physiological modelling sees changing patterns of mental and emotional conditioning towards sexual desire and appetite as tied to the same ageing process. The ageing process is considered 'naturally' and 'normally' desexualising, and exceptionalism represented as a departure often regarded as deviant (unless, for example, it conforms to stereotypes such as rampant male sexual appetite among socially successful men) (Simpson et al, 2023 *passim*).

The aesthetics of sex in later life is focused on the aesthetics of the ageing body in the context of a culture that produces and reproduces a 'premium' valuation of youthful and/or fit and healthy stereotypes and the potential 'ugliness' of ageing bodies (Moore and Reynolds, 2016). This aesthetic privileges representations of unblemished skin, unlined faces, taut bodies and features of youthful health reflecting stereotypes of sexual beauty and attraction, which can have some variance across different cultures and conjunctures.

Desexualisation conforms to a recognisable dominant sexual 'script' in relation to both the life course and sexual behaviours (what and when sex is 'normal' and 'natural'). The classical 'script' for sexual behaviours conforms to the Masters and Johnson (1966) linear sexual response cycle as a dominant paradigm for sexual pleasure – excitement, plateau, orgasm, resolution (though see critical alternatives such as Basson's (2001) circular model with a focus on women's responses). Here, genital stimulation is at the centre of sex. This in turn is the basis – not unqualified but still a basis – for a sexual hierarchy that privileges genito-centric heterosexual sex as defining 'normal' sexual pleasure. Genital centrality is oriented towards hierarchical models of sexual contact and more specifically towards a central notion of sex and pleasure that is functional, youthful, genital, penetrative, orgasmic (clitoral as well as penile) and intimate in bodily contact. This is explicit in the notion of 'normal' and 'natural' sexual practice and implicit in broader critiques of the dominant and hierarchical normativities of sexual identities, relations, orientations and behaviours. This scripting reinforces desexualisation as a dominant discourse in later life.

This hierarchical modelling of sex and sexuality should not be regarded as singular or linear. Histories of sexuality outline core dominant discourses: 'naturalistic' historical notions of sex that elided notions of sexual (orgasmic) pleasure first with procreation (up until the late 19th and early 20th centuries); then with good health (from the mid-20th century); then with degrees of normatively prescribed 'legitimate' sexual pleasure (from the late 1960s); that extends from heteronormative sex to homonormative (the end of the 20th century) (Primoratz, 1999; Weeks, 2016; Weeks, 2017). These were reflected in the development of sexology as a progressive science through the late 19th and 20th centuries (indicatively Bland and Doan, 1998a, 1998b). Yet, studies of Victorian England underline that while these dominant discourses were not popularly challenged, beneath the surface different sexual pleasures were practiced, reflecting diversity as sexual hierarchy ripples downwards (indicatively, Mason, 1994; Mort, 2000). Today, in predominantly Western, tolerant societies with degrees of homonormativity and more fluid conceptions of sex, there are permissible differences and digressions within a similarly ordered spectrum of sexual repertoire – in the case of homonormative sexual practice, perhaps a greater clitoral and wider erogenous stimulation for lesbian sex, and a greater focus on anal penetration or mutual masturbation in gay sex. There remains, however, the traditional focus on the genital, the directly bodily and the conception of pleasure along an orgasmic sexual response cycle.

The composition of sexual 'scripts' can change according to different cultural contexts and conjunctures, with traditional practices and attitudes bleeding into and providing roots for dominant and/or conservative notions of 'good sex', while dominant notions are themselves absorbing new sexual sub-cultures as they emerge. For example, wider ages between sexual partners (often referred to as 'May–December' relationships) may be more accepted in patriarchal societies across the global South. Equally, new conceptions of casual sexual relations such as 'friends with benefits' and sexual openness through 'distributed commitment' may gain recognition and degrees of acceptance at the fringes of monogamous relationships (indicatively, Plummer, 2015; Fischer and Seidman, 2016 *passim*; Weeks, 2022).

Hence, there is a tension that is contextual and conjunctural, between the specific and particular sexual forms aligned to different cultures and practices in different times and spaces, and a globalising, hierarchical, dominant culture transmitting Western and commodified sexual values, understandings and notions of what is erotic, desirable and sexually satisfying. In considering both desexualisation and resexualisation it would be a mistake to regard the composition of sexual cultures as uniform in their hierarchical form. The analysis of desexualisation involves a recognition that much that is desexualising involves culturally constructed discourses of medicine, health and what constitutes 'normal/natural' sex, which arises from sexological sciences and life course studies, overlaying and absorbing or relegating more specific and local cultural conventions and life course assumptions in different societies (indicatively, Caplan, 1987 *passim*; Holmberg, 1998; Parker and Aggleton, 2006 pass*im*; and Rees, 2024 *passim*).

Understanding the structure and order of the hierarchy of dominant to peripheral forms of sex and sexuality are important in three respects. First, it represents a modelling that accurately represents how sexual permissiveness and restrictions ebb, flow and fix in regulatory and discursive regimes at particular times and places. It therefore provides the foundations for more sophisticated analysis that recognises the complex relations that balance particular sexual contingencies and constraints. This can be applied critically to the particular opportunities and repressive restrictions of sex in later life.

Second, it provides a foundation for how the desexualising discourses overlaying the genito-centric core of sex can be understood in the face of the apparent contemporary contradictions, particularly in the way commodification appears to encourage new and diverse sexual markets even as traditional values appear predominant (Hennessy, 2000).

Finally, and obversely, it provides a framework of theorising the terms of resexualisation as a construction and a strategy, of which kink, in this example, can play a role. This framing of a critical analysis that can underpin resexualisation occupies the first section of this essay and is important as it provides an underlying narrative structure for the later discussion of kink as alternative.

In exploring resexualisation in later life, it is perfectly legitimate to focus on and evaluate those initiatives that might extend sexual pleasure into later life – such as pharmaceutical, technological, cosmetic surgical and surrogate opportunities. They can be adapted from serving a script that benefits later life, though within a context of dominant culture that orients otherwise. It is no surprise, then, that this volume concentrates on interventions – physiological (pharmaceutical and technological) and cultural (online communications, cyber alternatives and cultural change) – that can both augment and disrupt that desexualising orthodoxy. Desexualisation (Simpson et al, 2023) and resexualisation (this volume) tend towards a common subject of enquiry – the 'sexed' body with a genito-centric focus. This suggests and allows the persistence of the 'proper' deportment for sex as the unincumbered (often naked) body, where clothing and cosmetics are for bodily enhancement and the tease and deferral of foreplay, and the hierarchy of bodily stimulation begins with pre-genital contact and moves through digital and oral genital stimulation to arousal and genital penetration to orgasm, as observed in the sexual response cycle. These 'mainstream' components of sexual orthodoxy are therefore both boundaries to sexual difference and terrains of struggle and experimentation.

The other side of augmenting sexual pleasure in later life is to regard resexualisation as requiring substantial subversion of orthodox sexual scripts, or at least their subsumption without privilege within radical alternative sexual politics and practice. There is a strong sense in which mainstream sexual 'scripts' – themselves constructions rather than natural phenomena – require subversion and alternative constructions in order to negate or reverse their restrictive and pathological regulatory regimes. This is particularly evident when focus moves from the individual opportunities older people might seek to explore and enjoy, to consider substantive political change that transforms societal and cultural sexual values, regulatory regimes and discursive constructions. It is this process of conceptualising alternatives, and exploring kink as alternative, that occupies this chapter.

Of charmed circles, outer limits and hegemonic power

The subversive approach to sex ruptures, plays with, adapts or rejects the genito-centric sexual response cycle orthodoxy that constitutes a dominant form, as typified in analyses such as Rubin's (2011a: 152) 'charmed circle' (see Table 5.1). Rubin's model contrasts dominant orthodoxies for sexual identity, relations, orientations, behaviours and practices. Rubin's charmed circle summarises traditional silos within which legitimate sex is constituted, as opposed to the 'outer limits' which are either matters enjoyed in strict privacy without public disclosure or acknowledgement, or are subject to pathology, prejudice and legal and cultural constraint. Rubin's model represents the balance of legitimate and illegitimate sexual distinctions as seen from Rubin's radical critique when first published in 1982. As indicated above, while this might address a general global set of distinctions, it will vary when focused on particular cultures and contexts and in different conjunctures. Such a model allows the extension of sexual performance and pleasure into later life, but within conventions that orient towards such sexual engagement being regarded as exceptional, private and peripheral, alongside mainstream prejudice and pathology, and a broad absence of public/political recognition. Exclusion and invisibility lead to an absence of redistribution of resources to enable sex in later life, so that much of what is possible to facilitate sex is consumed on a purely private basis, with marginal public support.

Rubin's charmed circle has already been used to explore the possibilities for sex in later life. Jones (2020) observes that such a focus shows transgression across the lines of 'charmed circle' and 'outer limits', for example in the possible uses of technological enhancement to sexual pleasure, and inversion where the traditional focus of reproduction and marriage alongside sex is no longer relevant. This leads Jones (2020: 1492) to note that 'we should add an "age" spoke to the wheel: the inner charmed circle might be "sex involving young or middle-aged adults" and the outer limits might be "sex

Table 5.1: An outline of Rubin's criteria for 'charmed circle' and 'outer limits' represented in oppositional form with critical notes

Rubin's charmed circle	*Critical notes*	*Rubin's outer limits*
Good, normal, natural, blessed sexuality	Represented as opposites and not gradients/degrees	Bad, abnormal, unnatural, damned sexuality
Heterosexual	Exclusions – bi or queer	Homosexual
Married		Unmarried
Monogamous	Pejorative opposites – promiscuous not polyamorous	Promiscuous
Procreative	Cultural conventions that belie personal choice and mapping – married sadomasochist	Non-procreative
Non-commercial		Commercial
In pairs		Alone or in groups
In a relationship		Casual
Same generation		Cross-generational
In private		In public
No pornography		Pornography
Bodies only		With manufactured objects
Vanilla	Representative of its time	Sadomasochistic

involving children or old people"'. In doing that, she quickly qualifies that further 'spokes' to the wheel could be added (one is disability and difference in global cultures) that show the limits to the charmed circle as a means of distinguishing 'good and healthy' sex, and opens up critical discourses that lead to questioning its efficacy in the way Rubin suggests. Indeed, Rubin (2011b: 222–3) comments on the possible politics of how her analysis opened up and troubled norm/deviance distinctions in a reflection on her original essay 25 years later:

> One aspect of the essay of which I am most proud is its 'proto-queerness'. I wanted to move the discussion of sexual politics beyond single issues and single constituencies, from women and lesbians and gay men to analyses that could incorporate and address with more intricacy the cross-identifications and multiple subject positions that most of us occupy … I continue to believe that our best political hopes for the future lie in finding common ground and building coalitions based on mutual respect and appreciation of differences, and that the best intellectual work is able to accommodate complexity, treasure nuance, and resist the temptations of dogma and oversimplification.

Barker (2012) provides a more recent subversive alternative, where the charmed circle is given to plastic, fluid and enabling sexual characteristics over traditional, constraining and orthodox values. This model rejects the compulsory, singular and fixity of sexual convention, but not as necessity its components – so monogamy, for example, might be criticised as a norm but not as a chosen and adopted sexual choice. Its character is primarily contingent, plastic in the malleability of choices and enabling in sexual agents' composition of their own sexual 'scripts', while encouraging public openness, recognition and respect for sexual cultures that do not harm (see Table 5.2).

While the question of degrees of redistribution of public resources to enable diverse sexual choices are open questions, there is a tendency for those arguing for radical alternatives to focus on education, media as open space public debate and sexual literacy as means of enabling individuals and encouraging wider debate (Herdt et al, 2021; Moore and Reynolds, 2021; Reynolds, 2023).

Considering a more critical and political analysis, Raymond Williams (2005) provides a structure for understanding the relationship between residual (past), dominant (present) and emergent (future) cultures in the composition of contemporary sexual culture (Figure 5.1). Williams' model provides a significant advantage in how it represents contemporary cultural dominance. It understands is never static or complete but always in motion and therefore can be subject to disruption and change. This again speaks to the cultural construction of desexualisation and resexualisation.

Table 5.2: Barker's 2012 revision of Rubin's charmed circle/outer limits represented in contrast form with critical notes

Barker's charmed circle	*Critical notes*	*Barker's outer limits*
Consensual, critically informed, fluid, diverse sexuality	Represented in contrast and not gradients/degrees	Non-consensual, unaware, singular, fixed sexuality
Gender not necessarily relevant	Does not address mediated points that may be problematic, such as homonormative limits	Must be within heterosexual matrix (M/F self with M/F partner)
Can be within any relationship/no people/alone		Must be coupled romantic relationship
Consensual for all involved	'Fifty shades' BDSM that redraws legitimate/ illegitimate boundaries	Non-consensual, not communicated about or negotiated
May or may not involve physical contact		Focused on specific (genital) acts
May or may not have specific end point	The task of personal choice and mapping – sexual agency – remains, so the whole is as important as the sum of parts, so negotiated agentic spaces	Must lead to orgasm
All roles possible not necessarily gendered		Fixed gender roles (M – active/ initiating performing, F– passive receiving denying)
Desires and meanings differ within and between people		Universal: everyone must have the same sexual preferences
Critically informed and aware	Someone abstract charmed circle in order to maximise contingent positions but this may prove difficult unless adequate sexual literacy is achieved	Unaware of power dynamics and histories of privilege/oppression which may be in play
Fluid amount/type of desires shifts		Fixed and static sexual preferences
Diverse: any person/practice can be involved	Someone more specific outer limits that might pathologise legitimate choices, even if not intended	Narrow range of bodies/people/ relationships/acts can be sexual (others dysfunctional and abnormal)
Not imperative: May not be sexual		Imperative: individual and romantic relationships must be sexual
No fixed acceptable amounts/acts	Representative of its time and inherently political as well as public	Not too much or too little: certain activities must be/ must not be sexual (involving pain/power)

Figure 5.1: Williams' (2005) model of residual, dominant and emergent culture adapted for sexual culture

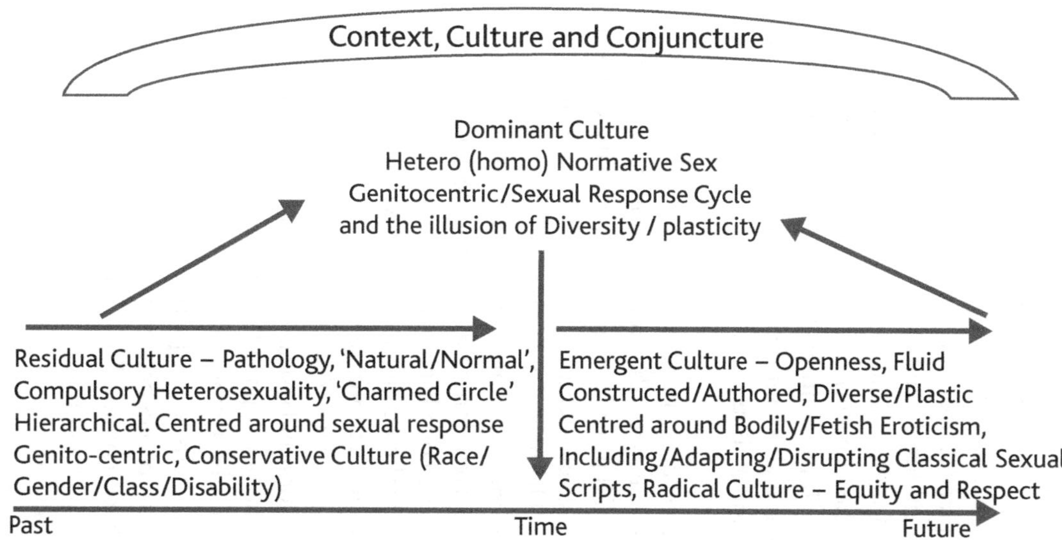

Figure 5.1: Context, culture and conjuncture

Williams (1977: 112–13) frames this through the concept of hegemony and the strategic maintenance of the status quo through a blend of coercion and consent. As Williams observes:

> A lived in hegemony is always a process. It is not, except analytically, a system or a structure. It is a realised complex of experiences, relationships, and activities, with specific and changing pressures and limits. In practice, that is, hegemony can never be singular. Its internal structures are highly complex, as can readily be seen in any concrete analysis. Moreover, (and this is crucial, reminding us of the necessary thrust of the concept), it does not just passively exist as a form of dominance. It has continually to be renewed, recreated, defended and modified. It is also continually resisted, limited, altered, challenged by pressures not at all its own.

Hegemony provides a framework that joins the everyday choices to explore sexual difference with the political impetus towards social change and transformation. It provides a means of conceiving explorations of and beyond 'conventional' genito-centric sex. It underlines the need for plurality, plasticity and diversity. The necessity of plurality and diversity explains, for example, why Barker's criteria within her charmed circle are so abstractive, and this corresponds to discussions of what constitutes kink (as discussed later). Indeed, Rubin's modelling of what is mainstream and what is more pathologised is in part criticised for being infected by Western values and constructs and being insufficiently intersectional (indicatively Hoad, 2011) This tension between the specificity of sexual pleasures and practices and the regulatory rules and conventions – local and global – with which they are governed provides space that enables the development of sub-cultures and the processes of cultural disruptions and absorptions of everyday practice (Williams, 2005: 31–49).

For example, fetishwear, particularly leatherwear, tightly stretched over 'orthodox' 'sexy' bodies became progressively a feature of advertisements for perfume or 'racy' commodities from the end of the twentieth century – and particularly in the context of the domestication of BDSM in mainstream markets by the '50 Shades of Grey' phenomena in the decade from 2011 (more on this later). Suddenly, everyone must have a 'crop', a vibrator/dildo and a 'sexy outfit' as long as they are the ineffectual products of sex shops like Ann Summers, and of limited, mainly visual, appreciation in 'foreplay' or lesser supplements to the absence of a partner. This invariably lays bare contradictions between the absorption of difference into dominant sexual scripts and the possibilities that they will in turn encourage exploration and experimentation that subverts.

How far these emergent cultural practices, or the retrieval of residual practices for contemporary pleasure, reflect a dominant culture that is strict and limiting, or porous and allowing openings for less 'conventional' sexual practices to enter the mainstream, is an open question. These answers are found in specific cultural, conjunctural and contextual analyses. Certainly, incorporation or absorption does not tend to threaten the existing orthodoxy but supplements it and reproduces hierarchical order that absorbs to order gradual change. Arguably this is where, for example, pharmaceutical supplements to enable sexual performance in later life might be located. While the fulfilment of sexual pleasure and performance remains associated with 'core' genito-centric practices, wider sexual repertoires have extended sexual horizons and been normalised and domesticated, particularly with what is regarded as foreplay. Foreplay allows sexual experimentation to be incorporated into orthodoxy and not challenge genito-centric hierarchy as literally the climax to sexual pleasure. These might include: licking, sucking, using fingers, kissing, touching flesh, with the extension of erotic clothing, sex toys like vibrators and some of what are regarded as 'kinky' practices – spanking, using edible body coverings, binding hands or binding to a bed, flogging are brought into play as arousal before orgasm. At the start of the 21st century, this 'erotic' foreplay has an industry producing commodities that meet its demands and cultural approval for 'experimentation' as by-waters, as long as it does not disrupt the overarching sexual order.

Extant sexual cultures and what they offer in pleasure should not be assumed or responded to as being unequivocally negative, certain and universal in their prevalence, onset, impact and consequences. Undoubtedly Viagra, for example, has given some men and heterosexual and gay or bisexual partners considerable pleasure, even if it works within a patriarchal, heteronormative and sometimes traditional sexual script of the active male leading the passive female (or 'feminised' man). Nevertheless, exploring the resexualisation of older people's intimate and pleasurable lives has to consider the balance of pleasures and constraints that are constituted by these new developments. Even stripped of their inclusion within desexualising discourses, there are changes and effects that must be factored into sexual lives as people grow older, where penetrative sex, for example, may be more difficult or less frequent or pleasurable. Given the power of discourses of genito-centrism, orgasm focus and bodily focus in constructing sex and sexuality in present culture, care needs to be taken not to simply see all adaptations as inherently problematic for people facing issues of sexual pleasure in later life today. That said, exploring a broader, plural, diverse and 'plastic' approach to sex, disassembling/reassembling and relocating changes in a more constructive paradigm is important in approaching resexualisation politically.

BDSM, kink and challenging sexual orthodoxy

There is a cluster of sub-cultures and penetrations of the dominant 'mainstream' sexual culture that have the capacity to fragment hierarchy and subvert the orthodoxy of the sexual cycle. These can and do operate within a genito-centrist and extant gendered and sexual orthodoxy but equally can amend or transform the sexual script to incorporate different pleasures or positions. These both preserve and displace the essential or 'climax point' or even constitute sexual pleasures that downgrades or absents genito-centrism and sexual orthodoxy. Further, they can extend outside the sexual cycle or disregard the cycle and its naturalising and normalising assumptions altogether. More, they redefine the very description of what constitutes sex within broader sensuous and erotic descriptions. These diverse pleasures and the people who practice them are broadly subsumed under the nomenclature BDSM (Bondage and Discipline [BD], Dominance and Submission [DS], Sadism and Masochism [SM]). Often, they are recognised in catch-all fashion as forms of 'kink'.

BDSM is often understood by the main features of its practice, which might be seen as playing with pain (SM), power (DS) and role (BD) (for a breakdown of these components see Weiss 2011: vii–xii). It is also associated with a range of equipment and apparel to facilitate erotic pleasure and fulfil a range of what are regarded as sexual fetishes. That presentation of fetishes is deliberate and problematic though accepted – particularly in the commodity form – since the classic Freudian conception would suggest that a fixation or reification of an intermediate object ahead of a desired 'other' (Freud, 1950). Here, the fetishes involve the use of objects, scenarios, places and scripts that amend, subvert, reinforce or defer from the domination frame of genito-centrism and the sexual response cycle, by either deferral, displacement or intermediate compulsion and desire. BDSM has a number of definitions that touch upon and reflect different understandings and positions. These have moved from the traditional pathology of sadism and masochism in the *DSM-5-TR* (American Psychiatric Association, 2022) to more positive representations:

> BDSM describes a range of *consensual* relational/sexual dynamics and behaviors which may include power, control, sensation play, restraints, punishment, and more. There is much variation in the way people 'play'. For some, BDSM is a lifestyle, while others may only engage casually on the weekends. The foundation of BDSM is open communication with your partner and consent! (Wright, 2023)

> For Active D&Sers sadomasochism is a thoughtful and controlled expression of adult sexuality that holds the promise of intense intimacy and sharing. (Brame et al, 1997: 8)

> SM employs various techniques to put one partner, the submissive, in a position of helplessness and vulnerability, and the other, the dominant in a position of command and authority. Bondage, sensory deprivation, flagellation, verbal dominance, behavior modification and mind games are some of the tools the dominant uses to control the submissive and guide … through an erotic experience. (Miller and Devon, 1995: 4)

> In Gosselin and Wilson's view, consensual 'SM' is a '…mutually agreed sexual relationship of unbalanced power' … and not reducible to a defined set of behaviours. Therefore, a new definition was championed which describes consensual 'SM' as: 'A relationship giving rise to the sexual interaction of two or more people via a ritual whose outward appearance involves coercion, pain, restriction or suffering of some kind but which has been agreed upon, tacitly or overtly, between the parties concerned and may in reality involve none of these constraints'. (Beckmann, 2009: 43)

An authoritative explanandum for contemporary BDSM comes from Langdridge and Barker (2013: 12) and is worth quoting at length.

> Generally 'sadist', 'dominant', 'dom/domme', and 'top' are used for the person in the position of power or the one giving out the stimulation and 'masochist', 'submissive', 'sub', and 'bottom' are used for the person with less power or the one on the receiving end. A 'switch' is someone who takes both kinds of roles. Often the words 'dominant' and 'submissive' are used for more psychological SM (e.g., that involving humiliation or servitude) and 'top' and 'bottom' for more physical (e.g., that involving pain or other sensations), although there is also often overlap between the two. SM activity may be referred to as 'play' or a 'scene' and non-SM sex may be termed 'vanilla'. Sometimes those who take part in SM are referred to as SM practitioners, although others prefer terms like 'SMers', since many in the SM communities view SM as an identity they have whilst others see it as an activity they practice … As mentioned above, a key phrase adopted by very many people engaging in SM is SM as 'safe, sane and consensual' (SSC), describing the core conditions for SM play. More recently, use of the acronym RACK (risk aware consensual kink) has grown in popularity, in recognition of the fact that no activity is 100% safe.

The common factor for such a diverse set of constitutive scripts, assemblages and practices is probably anything that changes, however marginally, the classic sexual script. The vernacular of 'vanilla' for conventional sexual appetites is contrasted with 'kink' for those who have different and diverse desires as the main or part of their sex lives. This absence of a singular description other than what it is not tends to make the borders of what constitutes BDSM porous and encourages the more nebulous use of the affirmation 'kink'. Some BDSMers make the argument that it is an identity (Langdridge and Parchev, 2018) – a culturally constituted lifestyle that can be lived 24/7 or within particular social and community and domestic spheres of life, which is important for legal, social and political recognition, it is a porous and plural identity in its constitution. For some, BDSM begins and ends in the bedroom or in online networking, or in 'munches' or meetings with likeminded 'kinkster's', or occasional visits to BDSM club nights with the possibility of some public play. Hence kink, and the focus on BDSM as a set of plastic and diverse ways of relating and acting sensuously and erotically, defies definite description. This underlines the importance of both the hegemonic framing of sexual politics, the recognition of the fluidity and plasticity of cultural constructions of sex and sexual pleasure and appetite, and so the centrality of choice by sexual agents.

As Sisson (2007) observes, while BDSM has become a visible subculture, it has strong historical antecedents and the ensemble of practices and approaches to non-conventional sex, if they have been marginal and peripheral in the way they have operated below the mainstream. Their growing visibility in the last 60 years – from exceptional and often perverted practice to subculture – has changed the dynamics towards more of a challenge or promise as alternative to the mainstream. Kinky sexual practices can marginally or more profoundly subvert the 'normal' whether through the incorporation of particular singular practices into vanilla sex, such as 'golden showers' (pissing on a partner) or bondage restraint, or a larger cultural engagement with a repertoire of kink practices bringing multiple sensations, role and pleasures. It is their composition in specific relations (couples, group, public/exhibition), and from specific 'sessions' (in the bedroom, the club, private party or the dungeon, for example) through to 'lifestyle 24/7' agreements, that provides degrees of subversion against genito-centric normativity. Kink can vary from being an adjunct to conventional sex to being permanent and constant (but evolving) feature and focus of an eroticised life, colonising every facet. This is to underline both the lack of determinant specificity in particular practices and at the same time the paradigmic shift that BDSM can represent. It can be adjunct, adaptation, extension, alternative and terrain of struggle in the same moment, in its relation to conventional conceptions of sex and sexuality and the emphasis on sexual play and pleasure.

Kink: sex as play and pleasure in later life

So, what does it offer the resexualisation of later life? To begin with, it loosens, disrupts or breaks the hegemonic dominance of 'mainstream' orthodoxy in sex. Sexual function and dysfunction are less a key parameter and the sexual cycle less or not at all a defining paradigm for sexual pleasure. Reproduction, health and conformity to sex in its conventional social forms, such as monogamy or coupling no longer have essential relationships for sex as a pleasurable activity. These are not forms that are disqualified – they are simply not compulsory nor more valid than other pleasures as a focus.

Reproduction is tangential to kink sex. It may reflect part of a personal lifestyle choice to reproduce, but this has no necessary relationship to how people enjoy pleasure. Technological means such as *in vitro*, alternative arrangements such as surrogacy, or more communal arrangements of parenting offer choices in which the penetrative act is one of many. Likewise, health issues or disabilities are not framed as impediments to sexual pleasure if pleasure arises from activities that recast and eroticise these conditions, which may influence choices and play, but do not of necessity detract from sexual pleasure. Amputations, mobility issues, physical weaknesses all become conditions that are considered in making sexual choices, rather than seen as impediments to sexual choices. Insofar as they impede some sexual practices, they may suit others. Someone with limited or no sensory pleasure genitally may well enjoy protracted massage, corporal punishment or other sensory stimulation of other parts of the body, seen as erotic and erogenous. Sex swings, for example, can enable people whose lower bodies are weak or immobilised to have penetrative sex or to be erotically stimulated, or to engage in pain/pleasure, as can queening stools or restraints and frames for supporting the body, such as Andrew's Crosses.

Erotic activity can be slowed to allow such preparations in restraint and support, where they are part of the erotic experience as well as preparatory measures. The use of sex aids or burlesque teases can quicken, slow or defer sexual responsiveness, rather than follow the 'natural' allotted sexual response cycle. Erotic play that involves pain pleasure may, or may not, involve orgasm (or not on every occasion) to deal with those who have difficulties with achieving orgasm. Erection and lubrication as features of sexual physiology are not necessary and certainly not the singular focal point. While there are now technologies – pharmaceutical, such as Viagra and Cialis, or artefacts such as surgically implanted sex pumps that enable erection, and forms of lubrication that aid women post-menopause – to enable function, it is conditional to a wider repertoire of activities that give different pleasures. These become optional supplements rather than expected adoptions to extend 'sexual life'. Non penetrative or non-orgasmic eroticism that stimulates, such as consenting voyeurism, erotic massage, dressing up to stimulate, playing with pain in spanking or whipping or piercing with needles – erotic torture – can all be seen as complementary or alternatives, and sex becomes less defined by constants – such as genital stimulation – and more by plurality and difference. Whatever stage of age in relation to health, there are options and choices. In addition, the dislocation of health from sex, or the accommodation of sex as a part of all people's lives, including those with health issues, is enabling.

In this context, for example it seems more than reasonable that hospices and care homes for the very aged – 80/90+ – should provide the means whereby masturbation, mutual masturbation, sensual play, playing with pain/ pleasure or submission and dominance – as well as fucking – is not only an option but facilitated as chosen. This is not to ignore the complexities of providing care for those in late life, but it is to argue that there is scope to change and amend practices and facilities to widen choice. Health, then, becomes not simply a constraint and in an inverse relationship with 'good, healthy sex'. Instead, it becomes something to be subject to creative thinking, to eroticise different bodies and minds (mental health being as important as physical health or their absences), to a mindset of inclusion and enabling, to eroticising lives *as they are*, and not according to some ideal, convention or stereotypical body or being. Impediments become opportunities, and people are not erotically defined as their disabilities or illnesses (or age ranges) but as people with differences.

As these sexual possibilities are outlined and considered in their endless diversity of relationships, 'partners' and practices, two concepts do bear further consideration: pleasure and play. While sex has always been acknowledged as pleasurable, it has been characterised by degree as dangerous and morally and physically debilitating according to how much it strays from convention and how important in time and attention it is to a person's life. The public acceptance of pleasure in sex education and health literature only began to take its place in the 1950s in Britain, for example, and dwelling on sex for pleasure in itself was and still is regarded as licentious. While pleasure is now a clear feature of contemporary sexual culture, served by commodity markets to 'enhance' experience, bourgeois notions of suspicion and pathology against those with a significant interest in their sexual pleasure remains.

A central rationale for kink and BDSM practices is precisely the exploration of self and others through practices that bring pleasure. This includes practices that bring different types of sexual pleasure, which might include masochistic satisfaction with enduring pain or discomfort, or submissive satisfaction in meeting the wants or needs of others, or the self-satisfaction of either imposing strict discipline or having it imposed in respect of bodily, mental or emotional task, or engaging in sessions of overindulgence. In this sense, both lack and excess bring pleasure, pleasure arises both directly from others and from the 'intermediate' sexual objects that can bring pleasure with or without others. This emphasises choice and communication between sexual agents.

Here, the concept of play becomes important. Play conveys the mixture of pleasure, experimentation and fun. Here, diversity and plasticity live in the playful practices of exploring and enjoying pleasures and desires, where sexual agents of any age construct their sex lives accordingly to their changing capabilities, relationships and explorations. This does not detract from safeguarding imperatives and sexual regulation, but it does take those matters that are not transgressing consent, agency and choice and renders them contingent practices/play that is inclusive to all and focused on pleasure. That observed, Newmahr (2011: 8–9) elaborates the cultural and political importance of play:

> 'play' is a complex word. It references recreation and leisure and evokes a romantic sense of innocence and freedom from encumbrances ... play is not a simple pursuit. It requires a significant amount of education, both formal and informal. It is exhausting, often physically, emotionally, and psychologically. Play encompasses a wide range of leisure activities and intimate interactions. It is a hobby and a lifestyle rife with political, social, and sexual implications.
>
> On one level, the discursive connections between SM and theatre provide access to the ideological (and emotional) defense that SM is somehow not quite real. (SM interactions, for example, are also called 'scenes'.) From this perspective, SM is more easily understood as an all-encompassing lifestyle that represents liberation from the oppressive plight of the everyman and nurtures identities of marginality. This community is built around play, and it is through play that community identities are constructed, sustained, and nurtured.

Newmahr's (2011) elaboration of play as both application and exploration is important, insofar as it rejects any easy notion of play as frivolity of an absence of considered engagement. It also connects the play of kink with the contingent opportunities of community which can enable a political agenda alongside a personal agenda of sexual pleasure and enjoyment.

Conclusion: kink, resexualisation in later life and play

One important caveat: these creative choices, enabling and opportunities should not be seen as simply compensatory – no notion of hierarchy should be injected into the plurality and plasticity of kink. At the same time, there should not be a second assumption that these are somehow mandatory or developmental for older, ill, disabled or others. Some older people, into substantive older age, can vigorously fuck penetratively and enjoy that, as can ill people and disabled people. A greater awareness and different approach to those who have needs that require adaptation or different opportunities should not become a 'norm' that instantiates a different set of assumptions about particular sexual agents.

Equally, this enabling of choice and opportunity should not in any way be seen as prejudicial against those who are or become asexual or less interested in sex (these are not the same thing), or who on balance at different stages of their lives ascribe it different – lesser or greater – values. Enabling 'no thanks' is as important as enabling 'yes please'.

Further, BDSM should not be romanticised as always already sexual radicalism and difference. While it can be subversive, it can also reflect the conventional sexual orthodoxy of capitalist heteropatriarchy (see, for example, Thompson, 1994: 14–16), and the commodification of kink reinforces and operates significantly to ensure that the market for sex products is enlarged, even to the point of serving some still pathologised sexual practices. So, the sex shop flogger and furry handcuffs are incorporated, whereas the whip, the tight and secure constraints and vacuum beds to immobilise the body completely are 'beyond the pale' (Weiss, 2006).

Beckmann (2009: 2) rehearses the contradiction between working within and alternative in kink to the extant order well:

> the 'bodily practices' of consensual 'SM' and their practitioners have a lot of resources to offer that stand in stark contrast to the reductionism of decontextualized commodified 'kink' that is marketed in consumer society.
>
> While it is evident that elements of 'SM' and of fetish culture have become part of capitalist consumerism and thus of mainstream society … Capitalism's proliferatory imperative led to the commodification and proliferation of representations of 'sex' as well as 'kinky sex'.
>
> there occurred a 'mainstreaming' of 'sadomasochist' representations in the media as well as of BDSM [Bondage Discipline, Dominance and Submission, SadoMasochism] behaviour forms. Despite the positive side-effects of greater access to tools, outfits, clubs, and so on, that were triggered by this (s)exploitation of 'kink' for commercial benefits, this trend cannot in itself be interpreted as representing a greater understanding or openness for the whole variety of these 'bodily practices' as they remain selectively criminalized … the important existential, inter-relational and political dimensions of consensual 'SM' play are totally absent from public representation.

Turley (2024) represents this tension between a normalised form of BDSM sub-culture and the transgressive possibilities of kink which both offer acceptance and public visibility drawing a line that domesticates elements within a revised conventionality while marginalising others – and these are important to consider notwithstanding the legitimacy of personal taking of the opportunities entering 'mainstream' sexual cultures.

With those caveats acknowledged, the construction and strategic aims and resexualisation – to enable, to expand and to inform and support choice and agency – gain both a wider repertoire and a loosening of cultural constraint from kink. In a sense, this extends to all sexual agents, but the agents that occupy this text – people in later life – have a particular vulnerability that arises from the pernicious cultural constraints of their earlier sexual experience, which might not be all pervasive but certainly influences their openness to possibilities. While conventional sexual histories tend to see waves of public openings of sexual freedom as arising from the 1960s and 1970s, these are partial and limited (indicatively Weeks, 2000: 163–78). Hence it is not just that resexualisation is a challenge to existing cultural conventions and standards, but that they are ingrained in people whose sexual histories may have largely followed convention and may then find breaking free of embedded notions of sex and sexuality in later life difficult. Here, the issue of education in its broadest sense – and particularly lifelong learning – and of space for public discussion and spaces where exploration can be seen, heard and considered becomes critical (see, for example, Barker and Hancock, 2017). The impetus to inform and encourage requires not only recognition bur redistribution of resources – and a politics that encourages positive change. In the absence of such a politics, the actions and initiatives of academics in producing knowledge, community groups in making space, sub-cultural groups in including and enabling and even business in taking commercial advantage but nevertheless representing opportunity, becomes imperative. Rubin's and later Barker's revised 'charmed circle' and Williams's model of hegemony become important here because they describe not only how to decode the present cultural construction of sexuality, but they signpost the possible politics of counter-hegemony or dissolution of a desexualising sexual order. This underlines that there is a political agenda as well as an interpersonal one, and resexualisation is a cultural and political project that requires collective action as well as individual exploration. As Weiss (2011: 30–1, 229) observes, drawing from her ethnographic experience with communities in San Francisco:

> SM community, practice, and performance produce a conduit between individual and social bodies, a circuit between the subjective (private desire, identity, individual autonomy, fantasy) and the socioeconomic (public community, social reality, collectivity, social power). In these circuits, BDSM names the specific ways in which practitioners situate themselves within and simultaneously reproduce larger social

> relations: iterations of public and private, community and commodity, self-mastery and technology, identity and social hierarchy.
>
> SM is a social practice that links bodies and subjects, selves and communities, private desires and public politics. When we parse the circuits that sexuality creates between individuals and social relations … we see the dynamic relationship between subjects and social hierarchies. Such circuits are productive: they draw on and reproduce the social horizon against which subjects, communities, and political imaginations gain force and legibility. The complicated circuits put into place through SM sex connect the embodied subject and the social body through commodity exchanges, through creative embodiments, through the ambivalences of gender and sex, and through the hierarchies of racial visibility. Not always subversive nor always capitulative, these exchanges *are* always productive; performances both depend on and produce material relations.
>
> Bauer (2014: 239) suggests that kink can bring about a sexual politics of 'exuberant intimacy' as a 'social space of excess, abundance and exuberance':
>
> Historically, excess has been the antidote to reason, and a judgment of excessive sexuality has been assigned to those who were constructed as irrational … excessive erotic practices, like dyke + queer BDSM, with its focus on boundary transgression, intensity and pleasure for its own sake, as well as its eroticization of everyday social worlds, may serve to disrupt the hegemonic notions of reason and sanity … these practices also reject enlightened and modernist imaginings of relationships as egalitarian or 'pure' … These non-innocent forms of social relations, which do not fall prey to the myth of equality … but, rather, acknowledge the ubiquity of power dynamics, may lead to acknowledging one's own social positions and one's emotional investments in them, such as eroticizing power relations. At the same time, they may provide access to excesses of sexualities that may be used productively to infuse socially devalued practices with erotic value and to create desires for subjugated and subversive social positions, not in the sense of eroticizing one's own oppression, but of imagining and experiencing spaces beyond hegemonic values and subject positions.

Where does this leave resexualisation and kink for later life? It situates an older population who face the orthodoxy of desexualisation with two interrelated pathways. The first, personal, incremental and tentative perhaps, yet full of promise, is to explore possibilities as sexual agents. Here kink offers a wider range of opportunities that can both compensate for reduced capacities as necessary but also provide new and different pleasures to add to their erotic experience. There, technology, pharmaceuticals and an availability of a wider range of sexual commodities can be of benefit, and individual agents determine the extent to which they incorporate such pleasures into their intimate lives. At the same time, these are always likely to be 'against the grain' of mainstream orthodoxy, with all the limits and constraints that involves.

As this becomes clear, there will be an impetus towards a second pathway, seeking change at collective and community levels, particularly with the resources of kink often situated in networks and cultural and social spaces. This politicisation, and a shift to seeking recognition and redistribution that enables kink and dissembles the present hegemony, may not be attractive to all sexual agents and the task of those who see the opportunities change offers and the resistance to forms of exploitation and oppression in sexual relations and practices is to seek to mobilise wider support for such change. Preferably these 'micro' and 'macro' trajectories will resonate together, though that is by no means to be assumed. In both cases, where resexualisation is a marginal pleasure or a substantive and existential change, kink offers much. What it also offers, above other incremental and individual opportunities, is a potential political framing that can be embraced as advancing a more creative, transformative and empowering sexual and social culture.

References

American Psychiatric Association (2022) *The Diagnostic and Statistical Manual of Mental Disorders* (5th edn) (DSM-5-TR), American Psychiatric Association Publishing.

Barker, M.-J. (2012) *Rubin Revisited: Rewriting the Rules* [online], Available from: https://www.rewriting-the-rules.com/sex/rubin-revisited/?subscribe=success#subscribe-blog-blog_subscription-2

Barker, M.-J. and Hancock, J. (2017) *Enjoy Sex: A Practical and Inclusive Guide*, Icon Books.

Basson, R. (2001) Human sex-response cycles, *Journal of Sex & Marital Therapy*, 27: 33–43.

Bauer, R. (2014) *Queer BDSM Intimacies: Critical Consent and Pushing Boundaries*, Palgrave Macmillan.

Beckmann, A. (2009) *The Social Construction of Sexuality and Perversion: Deconstructing Sadosmasochism*, Palgrave Macmillan.

Bland, L. and Doan, L. (1998a) *Sexology Uncensored: The Documents of Sexual Science*, Polity.

Bland, L. and Doan, L. (1998b) *Sexology in Culture: Labelling Bodies and Desires*, Polity.

Brame, G.G., Brame, W.D. and Jacobs, J. (1997) *Different Loving: The World of Sexual Dominance & Submission*, Century Press.

Caplan, P. (ed) (1987) *The Cultural Construction of Sexuality*, Routledge.

Fischer, N.L. and Seidman, S. (2016) *Introducing the New Sexuality Studies* (3rd edn), Routledge.

Freud, S. (1950) 'Fetishism' [1927], in J. Strachey (ed) *Sigmund Freud Collected Papers Volume 5*, Hogarth and Institute of Psycho-Analysis (1924–50), pp 198–204.

Hennessy, R. (2000) *Profit and Pleasure: Sexual Identities in Late Capitalism*, Routledge.

Herdt, G., Marzullo, M. and Petit, N.N. (2021) *Critical Sexual Literacy: Forecasting Trends in Sexual Politics, Diversity and Pedagogy*, Anthem Press.

Hoad, N. (2011) Rethinking sex from the Global South Africa, *GLQ: A Journal of Lesbian and Gay Studies*, 17(1): 119–24.

Holmberg, C.B. (1998) *Sexualities and Popular Culture*, Sage.

Jones, R. (2020) Later life sex and Rubin's 'charmed circle', *Sexuality and Culture*, 24: 1480–98.

Langdridge, D. and Barker, M. (eds) (2013) *Safe Sane and Consensual: Contemporary Perspectives of Sadomasochism*, Palgrave Macmillan.

Langdridge, D. and Parchev, O. (2018) Transgression and (sexual) citizenship: the political struggle for self-determination within BDSM communities, *Citizenship Studies*, 22(7): 667–84.

Mason, M. (1994) *The Making of Victorian Sexuality*, Oxford University Press.

Masters, W. and Johnson, V. (1966) *Human Sexual Response*, Little, Brown.

Miller. P. and Devon, M. (1995) *Screw the Roses, Send Me the Thorns: The Romance and Sexual Sorcery Of Sadomasochism*, Mystic Rose Books.

Moore, A. and Reynolds, P. (2016) Against the ugliness of age: towards an erotics of the aging sexual body, *Inter Alia*, 11a [online], Available from: http://interalia.org.pl/media/11A_2016/moore_reynolds.pdf

Moore, A. and Reynolds, P. (2021) Advocating sexual literacy, in: G. Herdt, M. Marzullo and N.N. Petit (eds) *Critical Sexual Literacy: Forecasting Trends in Sexual Politics, Diversity and Pedagogy*, Anthem Press, pp 323–32.

Mort, F. (2000) *Dangerous Sexualities: Medico-Moral Politics in England since 1830* (2nd edn), Routledge.

Newmahr, S. (2011) *Playing on the Edge: Sadomasochism, Risk, and Intimacy*, Indiana University Press.

Parker, R. and Aggleton, P. (eds) (2006) *Culture, Society and Sexuality: A Reader*, Routledge.

Plummer, K. (2015) *Cosmopolitan Sexualities*, Polity.

Primoratz, I. (1999) *Ethics of Sex*, Routledge.

Rees, E. (ed) (2024) *The Routledge Companion to Gender, Sexuality and Culture*, Routledge.

Reynolds, P. (2023) Consent and sexual literacy for older people, in P. Simpson, P. Reynolds and T. Hafford-Letchfield (eds) *Desexualisation in Later Life: The Limits of Sex and Intimacy*, Policy Press, pp 17–33.

Rubin, G. (2011a) 'Thinking sex: notes for a radical theory of the politics of sexuality', in *Deviations: A Gayle Rubin Reader*, Duke University Press, pp 137–81.

Rubin, G. (2011b) 'Blood under the bridge: Reflections on "thinking sex"' in *Deviations: A Gayle Rubin Reader*, Duke University Press, pp 194–223.

Simpson, P. (2015) *Middle-Aged Gay Men, Ageing and Ageism: over the Rainbow?* Palgrave Macmillan.

Simpson, P., Reynolds, P. and Hafford-Letchfield, T. (2023) *Desexualisation in Later Life: The Limits of Sex and Intimacy*, Policy Press.

Sisson, K. (2007) Heterosexual and bisexual S/M: cultural formations in G. Herdt and C. Howe (eds) *21st Century Sexualities: Contemporary Issues in Health, Education And Rights*, Routledge: pp 154–6.

Thompson, B. (1994) *Sadomasochism*, Cassell.

Turley, E. (2024) Unperverting the perverse: sacrificing transgression for normalised acceptance in the BDSM subculture, *Sexualities*, 27(9): 979–97.

Weeks, J. (2000) *Making Sexual History*, Polity.

Weeks, J. (2016) *Sexuality and Its Discontents: Meanings Myths and Modern Sexualities*, Routledge.

Weeks, J. (2017) *Sex, Politics and Society: The Regulation of Sexuality Since 1800* (4th edn), Routledge.

Weeks, J. (2022) *Sexuality* (5th edn), Routledge.

Weiss, M.G. (2006) Mainstreaming kink: the politics of BDSM representation in US popular media, *Journal of Homosexuality*, 50(2–3): 103–32.

Weiss, M. (2011) *Techniques of Pleasure: BDSM and The Circuits of Sexuality*, Duke University Press.

Williams, R. (1977) *Marxism and Literature*, Oxford University Press.

Williams, R. (2005) Base and superstructure in Marxist cultural theory [1973] in *Culture and Materialism*, Verso, pp 31–49.

Wright, S. (2023) BDSM: meaning, benefits and tips from a sexual therapist, in *Choosing Therapy* [online], Available from: https://www.choosingtherapy.com/bdsm/

PART II

Technologies and practices of resexualisation

6

Pharmaceutical culture and the resexualisation of later life

Barbara L. Marshall

> To come in to a doctor and say: I am losing (or I have lost) my sexual power, I wish you would give me some prescription for it ... which so many poor patients do, shows only the unsophisticatedness of the layman and his boundless belief in the miraculous power of medicine.
>
> Robinson, 1930: 159

> For the generation that refuses to grow old, Viagra is the drug everyone has been waiting and praying for. The pill that promises a lifetime of great sex – for just about everyone.
>
> Whitehead and Malloy, 1999: 2

> Now you can have sex when, where, and how you want it, dependably and reliably, even if you're 100 and your partner's 102.
>
> Vaughn, 1998: 14

As the epigraphs suggest, there has been a sea-change in popular understandings of sex, ageing and the 'miraculous power of medicine'. The pharmaceutical resexualisation of later life lauded here, with a starring role for Viagra, is part of a broader shift in understandings of the role of sexual activity in what constitutes healthy and 'successful' ageing. Eli Coleman, former president of the World Association for Sexology, links this 'new sexual revolution' to increased longevity:

> people are living longer. Consequently, they are sexually active longer. This has created a demand to help older people function sexually. Science has responded with more research to understand the sexuality and ageing process and to develop ways of keeping people sexually active through biomedical interventions ... For men and women alike, ageing will no longer signal the retirement of sexual behaviours. People will now be able to maintain virility and sexual activity much longer. (Coleman, 1999/2000: 5)

Coleman's summary echoes the progress story told by sexual medicine, one underpinned by the dominance of biomedical models of sexual function and culminating in the triumph of sexuopharmaceuticals (Goldstein and Goldstein, 2024).

Sexuality, especially where older people are concerned, has become increasingly medicalised, and the pharmaceutical industry has been influential in this process. Medicalisation, or the process by which common experiences and discontents become understood as medical diagnoses, has long been an important concept in the social sciences. While early critiques focused on the extension of medical professionals' control over ordinary people (Illich, 1976), more recent approaches have identified commercial and market interests as playing an increasingly important role (Conrad, 2005). A global pharmaceutical industry has invested massively in the development of drugs, the delineation of conditions that they might treat and the marketing of both diagnoses and remedies. As summarised by Jutel and Mintzes (2018): 'The drivers of medicalisation are increasingly positioned outside of medicine, issuing instead from the pharmaceutical and biotechnology industries and from the patient-consumer, primed by these commercial entities to consider themselves in need of medical support' (162). The dissemination of health information through the internet, direct to consumer advertising, and pharmaceutical industry promotion of specific conditions through clinical education and construction of diagnostic and clinical guidelines all contribute to medicalisation and pharmaceuticalisation (Bergey, 2018).

In contrast to the linear model of scientific progress that underpins the dominant discourse around the pharmaceutical resexualisation of later life, this chapter argues that there is a more complex story to be told. While diagnoses of sexual dysfunctions are often presented as 'facts of nature' which have been 'discovered' through the diligent labour of scientists, they 'hide a deeply grounded, socially negotiated genesis' (Jutel, 2011: 2). In other words, they do not just rest on medical fact, but reflect some sort of social agreement about the undesirability of a condition that demands treatment.

This chapter highlights resexualisation as encompassing not only the process whereby pharmaceutical technologies are designed to eliminate ageing as a barrier to youthful levels of sexual function and performance, but also the ways in which these are framed in distinctly gendered and heterosexist ways. Pharmaceutical resexualisation is premised on an understanding of sexual activity framed by a reproductive model that has penetrative intercourse at its centre, contributing to a problematic and reductive conceptualisation of what constitutes the 'sex' in resexualisation.

The chapter begins with an historical review of medicine's interest in late-life sexuality and the shifting aetiologies of sexual disorders over the 20th century. It then turns to the pivotal role that the introduction of erectile medications such as Viagra played in revising conceptualisations of sexual life courses, including the broader medicalisation and pharmaceuticalisation of sexual desire and function in both men and women. After discussion of the cultural narratives that provide critical framing for the pharmaceutical resexualisation of later life, conclusions ponder how these might be the focus of critique and revision to nurture more inclusive and expansive resources for navigating sexuality across the life course.

From decline to dysfunction

Medical understandings of sexuality in later life have shifted dramatically since the turn of the 20th century, when it was widely assumed that both men and women in midlife faced a 'climacteric', ushering in a post-sexual (and potentially androgynous) later life (Marshall and Katz, 2006). Common wisdom praised the benefits of this transition, and individuals were counselled to accept this with graceful adjustment. After all, sexual life was tied to reproductive life, making sexual decline an expected part of ageing. However, as the hormonal model of differently sexed bodies was stabilised, rejuvenation science and developments in endocrinology held out the promise of intervention (Oudshoorn, 1994; Roberts, 2002; Sengoopta, 2006).

While belief in the inevitability of sexual decline persisted well into the 20th century, it was challenged by those who believed the sex glands held the secret to revitalisation (Marshall, 2020). Masculinity was especially tied to the 'internal secretions' of the testicles and attempts to rejuvenate men through various experiments with testicular transplants, injections and surgeries to permit the reabsorption of testicular fluids gained notoriety through the 1920s. Yet the restoration of sexual virility was not the primary goal of rejuvenation enthusiasts, who were more concerned with shoring up masculine productivity. Instead, resexualisation cast a pall of immorality over the whole enterprise, which its defenders sought to counter with reminders of the other benefits, like increased energy for work. Less common rejuvenation attempts with women were even less tied to sexuality. Harry Benjamin, the best-known practitioner, reported to the World Sex Reform Congress in 1929 on the results of several hundred cases of females treated with hormones and/or x-ray stimulation of the ovaries and pituitary gland, noting that the restoration of sexual potency 'plays very rarely a part in the mind of the ageing woman. Much more often a cosmetic effect is desired' (Benjamin, 1929: 565).

While rejuvenation experiments were largely discredited by the 1930s, their legacy was not inconsequential. As Susan Squier commented: 'They generated controversy in the popular press, became the focus of best sellers, canonical novels and science fiction short stories, provided the theme for a smash Hollywood movie and exercised a shaping impact on our attitudes toward ageing that persist to the present day' (Squier, 1999: 89). The 'attitudes' alluded to here are, of course, those that grounded the conviction that science can transform the ageing process.

The most important cultural legacy of early endocrinology was the 'fundamental assumption that sex hormones are essential for the maintenance of health, well-being, libido and general vitality' (Sengoopta, 2001: 645). Estrogen and testosterone were seen as the very essences of femininity and masculinity, whose ebb and flow came to define sexual life courses. As Gullette summarises it: 'Their minuscule chemical traces gave the world a major metaphor for difference between youth and age and between men and women' (2003: 73). By the 1930s, both estrogen and testosterone were being synthesised in laboratories and offered up as interventions against the desexualisation of ageing bodies.

By the 1960s, hormone replacement therapy (HRT) was promoted as something all women should consider for the entirety of their post-menopausal life, especially through popular works like *Feminine Forever* (Wilson, 1966) which argued that without estrogen, women would be neutered by the ageing process. The idea of a hormonally based 'male climacteric', analogous to the female menopause and, like the latter, treatable with HRT, also gained traction in the 1930s and 1940s. However, by the 1950s, it had virtually disappeared from the medical literature. Instead, men's complaints were re-framed as a stress-related midlife syndrome, and the therapeutic regime shifted from testosterone to tranquilisers (Watkins, 2008). Men continued to worry about their erections, but psychological explanations for mid to later life impotence gained the upper hand. As summarised by the *Encyclopedia of Love and Sex* in 1972: 'The most common cause of the loss of sexual ability in the older man is mental negativism and fear, rather than physical degeneration' (Fletcher, 1972: 164). The toolkit of remedies now included counselling, lifestyle modifications and, where warranted, mechanical devices such as vacuum pumps and penile prostheses.

Developments in urology were taking a different direction, demonstrating the ability to induce a penile erection by purely *chemical* means. This set the stage for the development of new pharmaceutical therapies for impotence, such as penile injections and tablets inserted into the urethra. New disease models were constructed which weakened the link between sexual decline and 'normal ageing', suggesting that 'modifiable para-ageing phenomena' were the problem (Feldman et al, 1994).

In 1992, the US National Institute of Health convened a consensus conference on 'impotence' from which the first recommendation was a shift in terminology to 'erectile dysfunction'. The final report also concluded that 'the likelihood of erectile dysfunction increases with age but is not an inevitable consequence of ageing', offering instead that 'many cases of erectile dysfunction can be successfully managed with appropriately selected therapy'.

Erectile dysfunction is, the report stressed, 'an important public health problem deserving of increased support for basic science investigation and applied research' (National Institute of Health, 1992: 28–9). Its prevalence was anticipated to increase as populations aged, with intimations that an epidemic could be on the horizon (Aytac et al, 1999).

Frequently cited to establish the age-related incidence of erectile dysfunction (ED) was the Massachusetts Male Aging Study (McKinlay and Feldman, 1994), based on a random sample of men between 40 and 70 years of age studied over a 2-year period. However, missing from the ubiquitous citations to this study supporting claims of a pending epidemic and the urgent need for medical remedies, was the finding that increased incidence of erectile problems with age did not necessarily mean distress for men. To the contrary, 'despite the marked declines in actual events and behaviour and in subjective aspects of sexuality, men in their sixties reported levels of satisfaction with their sex life and partners at about the same level as younger men in their forties' (McKinley and Feldman, 1994: 272). The pharmaceutical industry had a stake in actively re-orienting these normative expectations and did so with overwhelming success in the development and marketing of sexuopharmaceuticals – none more so than with Viagra.

Viagra and after

Viagra – the brand name of sildenafil – is the best known of the sexuopharmaceuticals, sildenafil is a PDE-5 inhibitor, which enhances the smooth muscle relaxation that maintains blood flow to the penis. The story of Viagra's development and success has now been widely recounted (see, for example, Loe, 2004a; Tiefer, 2006; Fishman, 2010; Loeb et al, 2024). Approved by the US Food and Drug Administration (FDA) in 1998, it is one of the most commercially successful drugs on record. Viagra's success not only revolutionised the diagnosis and treatment of erectile difficulties but ensured the hegemony of a biomedical narrative of sexual ageing. As one prominent researcher summarised: 'Baseless speculation about the essential vascular mechanisms of erection and the belief in a predominantly emotional etiology have given way to the identification of molecular events resulting in an erection and to effective pharmacological treatment of their alterations' (Morales, 1998: xv). Viagra was presented as the solution to a rather simple mechanical problem. As explained by urologist Irwin Goldstein: 'The man needs a sufficient axial rigidity so his penis can penetrate through labia, and he has to sustain that in order to have sex. This is a mechanical structure, and mechanical structures follow scientific principles' (as cited by Hitt, 2000: 36). Goldstein's explanation here also underscores the reductive understanding of 'sex' as penetrative penile-vaginal intercourse, and that phallocentric and heterosexist framing was also reflected across the clinical research and marketing associated with the rollout of sexuopharmaceuticals (Mamo and Fishman, 2001; Marshall, 2002; 2010; Wentzell, 2011).

Viagra was both a pharmaceutical phenomenon, earning millions for Pfizer, and a cultural phenomenon, even warranting an entry in the Oxford English Dictionary within just a few years (Oxford English Dictionary, 2001). Viagra's cultural take-up has been rife with hyperbole. It has been called a 'miracle drug' (Jarow et al, 1998), a 'wonder drug' (Whitehead and Malloy, 1999) and seen as defining a new age, speculating that 'we may one day come to designate everything that has happened prior to April 1998 as "before Viagra" and everything since "after Viagra"' (Melchiode and Sloan, 1999: 228). Its impact also prompted academics to take up 'Viagra studies' (Tiefer, 2006), exploring life in the 'era' of Viagra (Vares et al, 2007; Ferrero Camoletto, 2019), its role in grounding new forms of identity and personhood (Stock and Moser, 2001; Potts, 2005; Asberg and Johnson, 2009; Johnson et al, 2011), and critically exploring the 'Viagrisation' of sexual discontents (Castro-Vazquez, 2006; Ferrero Camoletto et al, 2020).

There is no question that Viagra heralded a sea change in understandings of sexual life courses, especially for men. As one of the many mainstream press articles reflecting on its history noted, 'it transformed a private frustration for many ageing men into a publicly discussed medical condition with an easy treatment' (Johnson, 2017). Another remarked that Viagra's success, alongside the introduction of other erectile drugs a few years later, 'ushered in a decade when it was nearly impossible to avoid commercials for drugs promising to improve the sex life of middle-aged men' (Quartz staff, 2018). Erectile drugs that followed Viagra onto the market include Levitra (Vardenafil), Cialis (Tadalafil) and Stendra (Avanafil), with all but Stendra now available in generic forms as patents have expired. While existing erectile medications do not work well for everyone, and there is evidence that their efficacy may decrease with long-term use, the promise of a lucrative and ever-growing market continues to stoke pharmaceutical industry interest in the development of future medications (Cox, 2019). It has also mobilised interest in other drugs – both those such as testosterone, related to a broader medicalisation of older men's sexuality, and those targeting women as a potentially huge untapped market.

As noted earlier, the concept of a hormonally treatable male menopause had waned by the mid 20th century, with the sexual discontents of ageing men cast as more psychological than physical in origin. However, the pharmaceutical resexualisation of ageing men in the late 1990s involved more than Viagra. As one newspaper article on men's health in midlife warned its readers who may have thought erections were their only problem: 'If you think you can Viagra your way out of this one, think again: It and similar drugs might help with the mechanics, but not with desire; testosterone is what fires the libido' (Werland, 2004: 9). Viagra's success, along with new delivery methods for testosterone, such as transdermal gels and patches, rejuvenated biomedical and industry interest in the idea of 'andropause' as a treatable hormone deficiency for which a decline in sexual interest and performance was a key indicator. The term 'andropause' was replaced by the more clinical 'Androgen deficiency in the aging male' (ADAM) (Wyllie, 2003), and subsequently 'Late onset hypogonadism' (LOH) (Morales, 2008). LOH is defined first and foremost by: 'The easily recognised features of diminished sexual desire (libido) and erectile quality and frequency' (Nieschlag et al, 2005: 56).

In addition to sexual complaints, a diagnosis of LOH links other symptoms, such as decreased muscle mass, increased body fat and decreased energy to a 'deficiency in serum testosterone levels (below the young healthy adult male reference range)' (Wang et al, 2008: 508), effectively associating full masculinity with the capacities of youth and casting age as a universal risk factor. The latter focus opened the door to claims that, should insurers refuse to pay for testosterone supplementation, they are 'ageist' and harbour a 'Victorian attitude towards sex' (Morley, 2007: 555). While diagnoses of LOH and the use of testosterone for the sexual complaints of ageing men remain controversial, robust marketing on the part of pharmaceutical companies has buoyed prescription rates (Bandari et al, 2017; Busnelli et al, 2017; Layton, 2017).

The medicalisation and pharmaceuticalisation of female sexual dysfunction have been less successful, less age focused and more problematic in their construction of disease categories than that of men. While HRT for women suffered a sharp drop after the Women's Health Initiative warned of potential health risks in 2002, the pharmaceutical industry made a concerted – and largely successful – effort to re-boost prescription rates for estrogen and progesterone (Fugh-Berman, 2015). While there has always been an undertone of resexualisation to the 're-feminising' discourse of HRT for women, the post-Viagra years have witnessed more explicit pharmaceutical attention to women's sexuality, focusing on the restoration of both women's desire for, and physical receptiveness to, penetrative sexual intercourse.

Before the 'hunt for pink Viagra' (Wyllie, 2005) took off in earnest, Viagra itself was tested on women, guided by the assumption that there were similar physiological actions at root. Because erectile medications targeted blood flow to the genitals, 'vasculogenic female sexual dysfunction' was constructed as a target through diagnoses such as 'vaginal engorgement and clitoral erectile insufficiency syndrome' (Goldstein and Berman, 1998). Despite repeated clinical trials, no benefit was demonstrated, and Pfizer stopped testing Viagra on women in 2004.

A crossover to women was also attempted with testosterone, with the hope of increasing sexual desire. A transdermal testosterone patch for women, Intrinsa, tested as a treatment for 'Female Androgen Insufficiency

Syndrome', failed to get approval in the US, but made it to market in the EU in 2006, only to be voluntarily withdrawn in 2012 for 'commercial reasons' (European Medicines Agency, 2012). Despite the fact that there are currently no approved testosterone supplements for women, they continue to be prescribed off-label, despite continuing debates about efficacy (Lowenstein et al, 2016; Islam et al, 2019).

The pharmaceutical industry also focused on drug development specifically aimed at women's desire deficit, and two products are now on the market in the US. Flibanserin, a failed anti-depressant marketed as a pink pill called 'Addyi', was approved by the FDA in 2015 as a treatment for 'hypoactive sexual desire disorder' in pre-menopausal women. Bremalanotide, an injectable melacortanin agonist marketed as 'Vyleesi' was approved in 2019, also for pre-menopausal women. Neither have replicated the commercial success of erectile drugs, no doubt in part due to their limited demonstrated benefits and numerous side-effects (Thangaraju et al, 2022; Spielmans and Ellefson, 2024). While neither is approved for post-menopausal women, anecdotally they are being prescribed off-label and trials with older women have begun (Portman et al, 2017; Goldstein et al, 2023), suggesting that an application to approve them for more specifically age-related decline in sexual desire may be forthcoming.

More clearly focused on a specific concern of many older women are remedies to address the thinning and drying of vaginal tissues. While topical treatments – such as vaginal moisturisers and hormone creams – have been available for many years, more recent pharmaceutical products have targeted not the general issues of genital pain or dryness, but specifically dyspaenuria, or painful intercourse. Osphena, for example, a selective estrogen receptor modulator, was approved by the FDA in 2013, and even though it shared no biological basis for comparison with Viagra, was lauded as a 'winner' in the 'race for a pink Viagra' (Cacchioni, 2015: 54). Restoring women's physical receptiveness to penetrative vaginal intercourse is seen as the primary benefit. As Bedor (2015) notes in her analysis of Osphena marketing, the cultural narratives deployed are not so much about women's own desires, but about women as being ready for sex with a partner – where 'sex' is understood as heterosexual intercourse.

Expanding the narrative framing of sex and ageing

A growing body of critical work on sexuopharmaceuticals, emphasising their relationship to cultural narratives of later life, provides a richer and more complex picture of ageing and sexuality than that which has underpinned the promotion of pharmaceutical resexualisation. Particularly important here are qualitative studies which have explored sexuopharmaceutical marketing, dispensing and use in different cultural contexts and with regard to diversity in users or potential users (Potts et al, 2003; Loe, 2004b; Asberg and Johnson, 2009; Bertone and Ferrero Camoletto, 2009; Erol, 2014; Ferrero Camoletto et al, 2015; Alarcão et al, 2016; Erol and Ozbay, 2017; Rohden, 2017; Rohden, 2019; Ferrero Camoletto, 2021; Wentzell, 2021). Despite the best efforts of pharmaceutical marketers, their products are not taken up uniformly or without active engagement on the part of users. For example, the initial rollout of Viagra as a medical technology to support heterosexual relationships characterised its use by gay men as 'recreational' and 'risky' (Wentzell, 2011). Yet Wallach et al (2020), for example, found that both gay and heterosexual older men expressed reasons for using erectile medications that deviated from the 'therapeutic objectives' of dominant pharmaceutical scripts, and that in practice, 'corrective' and 'enhancement' objectives were not mutually exclusive in the stories of men they interviewed. In another example, anthropologist Emily Wentzell's work in Mexico (Wentzell, 2013, 2017) demonstrates the uneven success of global pharmaceutical company attempts to export Western ideas of 'good' sexual ageing. She found that, while erectile drugs were widely promoted in Mexico, and on the surface might seem to be compatible with popular notions of 'machismo', a significant subset of the Mexican men she interviewed rejected their use. Instead, they drew on narratives of masculinities changing with age, with decreased erectile function perhaps even helping them to age *better*, in what they understood as more socially appropriate ways. For Wentzell (2021) this underscored the limits of the Western emphasis on individuality which under-emphasises the importance of relational contexts. Similarly, Ferrero Camoletto's research with Italian doctors (Ferrero Camoletto et al, 2015; Ferrero Camoletto, 2021) shows both the spread of a globalised pharmaceutical script for successful sexual ageing and some of the complexities of their local enactments. While some doctors upheld the framing of sexuopharmaceuticals as something suffering individuals had a 'right' to, many also believed that their patients' health would benefit more from 'age-appropriate' lifestyles. Even while generally endorsing a biological basis for sexual function and dysfunction, there were also moral lines to be drawn that complicated the pharmaceutical script.

In sum, while sexual medicine and a global pharmaceutical industry approach sexuality through a biomedical lens, corporealising and universalising understandings of sexual changes associated with age, qualitative research suggests that 'the same biological changes can be understood very differently in different contexts' (Wentzell and Labuski, 2020: 29). The contradictory alternatives of an asexual old age or the never-changing heterosexiness on offer through pharmaceutical narratives do not provide much of a range of positions for people to take up, nor do they resonate with what qualitative research has found about older peoples' experience (Tetley et al, 2018). It is particularly important, then, to highlight the cultural narratives that provide resources for understanding and experiencing sexuality across the life course, including decisions to use (or not to use) sexuopharmaceuticals.

The point of critiques of sexuopharmaceuticals such as Viagra is not to suggest that they should be rejected out of hand. Instead, as Kristina Gupta argues, 'we must change the social and cultural context' in which they are used (Gupta, 2019: 75). To this end, Gupta suggests challenging a host of cultural assumptions around sexuality, gender and race. Particularly relevant to critiques of the pharmaceuticalisation of later life sexuality are Gupta's calls to:

- challenge the notion that health and happiness are dependent on sexual activity;
- expand conceptions of sexual pleasure and fulfillment beyond the focus on penetrative intercourse;
- critique conventional 'scripts' of masculinity, femininity and heteronormativity that are tied to particular expressions of sexuality;
- critique the understanding of sexual difficulties as primarily organic and emphasise the important role of non-biomedical approaches (such as sex education and counselling) in addressing them. (Gupta, 2019)

In addition to these factors, there is a need to challenge more explicitly the assumptions of 'successful' ageing and 'anti-ageing', even when these are couched in the language of anti-age*ism*. Too often, these only thinly disguise novel forms of ageism – what has been called 'post-ageist ageism', where 'anti-ageist sentiments are embraced at the same time as old age is constructed as something to be resisted' (Marshall and Katz, 2012: 230). The promise of sexuopharmaceuticals to provide the proverbial fountain of sexual youth is both misleading and denigratory towards the embodied realities of 'living in time' (Katz, 2011: 188). It is particularly important, then, to critique claims that 'sexual rights in older age are synonymous with the right to access medical intervention to continue youthful and normative forms of sexuality' (Ferrero Camoletto et al, 2020: 126).

Conclusions

This chapter has argued that the pharmaceutical resexualisation of older people has been premised on important shifts in medical understandings of sexuality in later life. The disorders that problematise sexual ageing today would not have made sense a century ago, as cultural narratives have shifted in relation to available remedies.

The clinical and market success of erectile medications like Viagra has been instrumental in shaping the resexualisation of later life, and in forging new narratives of age-related sexual changes as pathological and pharmacologically treatable. Viagra has proven to be more than just a treatment for erectile dysfunction as it has revised expectations and normalised pharmaceutical intervention into sexual changes over the life course. The success of erectile medications spurred widespread interest in developing larger markets for sexuopharmaceuticals, including desire enhancers for women and hormonal treatments for men.

With age cast as a 'risk factor' for a range of sexual difficulties (now defined as dysfunctions or disorders) ageing populations in Western nations have prompted the pharmaceutical industry to argue that 'unmet medical needs in sexual dysfunction provide the necessary backdrop for therapeutic opportunities and advances' (Kim and Uhl, 2011: 4). In other words, changes in sexual desire and capacities might be expected with age, but as with other conditions (such as hypertension and presbyopia) they should be seen as treatable. However, as this chapter has argued, pharmaceutical resexualisation involves not only efforts to eliminate ageing as a barrier to sexual function and performance, but also the re-entrenchment of sex difference in gendered, heterosexist, ablest and ageist ways. It seems particularly important to underscore the ageism implicit in pharmaceutical resexualisation. As long as being sexualised means adhering to youthful norms of sexual attractiveness and prioritising sexual intercourse as the gold standard of sexual function, 'it is not old age that is being sexualised but rather an extended middle age. The incompatibility of sexuality and old age is hence reinforced' (Gott, 2005: 2).

As other chapters in this volume (and in other volumes in this series) have stressed, 'ageing' and 'sexuality' are complexly related through intersections of cultural narratives, social structures and material conditions. In this spirit, to be critical of pharmaceutical resexualisation is not to reject these technologies out of hand, but to consider how they might figure into the broader project of promoting a less reductive understanding of sexual rights and sexual agency for older people.

References

Alarcão, V., Machado, F.L. and Giami, A. (2016) Traditions and contradictions of sexual function definitions for Portuguese heterosexual men and women: medicalization and socially constructed gender effects, *Sexual and Relationship Therapy*, 31(3): 271–88.

Asberg, C. and Johnson, E. (2009) Viagra selfhood: pharmaceutical advertising and the visual formation of Swedish masculinity, *Health Care Analysis*, 17(2): 144–57.

Aytac, I.A., McKinlay, J.B. and Krane, R.J. (1999) The likely worldwide increase in erectile dysfunction between 1995 and 2025 and some possible policy consequences, British Journal of Urology International, 84: 50–6.

Bandari, J., Ayyash, O.M., Emery, S.L., Wessel, C.B. and Davies, B.J. (2017) Marketing and testosterone treatment in the US: a systematic review, *European Urology Focus*, 3(4): 395–402.

Bedor, E. (2015) It's not you, it's your (old) vagina: Osphena's articulation of sexual dysfunction, *Sexuality & Culture*, 20(1): 38–55.

Benjamin, H. (1929) The reactivation of women, in N. Haire (ed) *Third Congress of the World League for Sexual Reform*, Kegan Paul, Trench, Trubner and Co. Ltd, pp 564–73.

Bergey, M.R. (2018) The changing drivers of medicalisation, in B.M.Z. Cohen (ed) *Routledge International Handbook of Critical Mental Health*, Routledge, pp 153–61.

Bertone, C. and Ferrero Camoletto, R. (2009) Beyond the sex machine? Sexual practices and masculinity in adult men's heterosexual accounts, *Journal of Gender Studies*, 18(4): 369–86.

Busnelli, A., Somigliana, E. and Vercellini, P. (2017) 'Forever young' – testosterone replacement therapy: a blockbuster drug despite flabby evidence and broken promises, *Human Reproduction*, 32(4): 719–24.

Cacchioni, T. (2015) *Big Pharma, Women and the Labour of Love*, University of Toronto Press.

Castro-Vazquez, G. (2006) The politics of Viagra: gender, dysfunction and reproduction in Japan, *Body and Society*, 12(2): 109–29.

Coleman, E. (1999/2000) A new sexual revolution in health, diversity and rights, *SIECUS Report*, 28(2): 4–8.

Conrad, P. (2005) The shifting engines of medicalization, *Journal of Health and Social Behavior*, 46(1): 3–14.

Cox, D. (2019) The race to replace Viagra, The Observer [online] 9 June, Available from: https://www.theguardian.com/science/2019/jun/09/race-to-replace-viagra-patents-erectile-dysfunction-drug-medical-research-cialis-eroxon.

Erol, M. (2014) From opportunity to obligation: medicalization of post-menopausal sexuality in Turkey, Sexualities, 17(1–2): 43–62.

Erol, M. and Ozbay, C. (2017) No andropause for gay men? The body, aging and sexuality in Turkey, *Journal of Gender Studies*, 27(7): 847–59.

European Medicines Agency (2012) Public statement on Intrinsa, withdrawal of the marketing authorisation in the European Union [online], Available from: https://www.ema.europa.eu/en/documents/public-statement/public-statement-intrinsa-withdrawal-marketing-authorisation-european-union_en.pdf

Feldman, H.A., Goldstein, I., Hatzichristou, D.G., Krane, R.J. and McKinlay, J.B. (1994) Impotence and its medical and psychosocial correlates: results of the Massachusetts male aging study, *Journal of Urology*, 151: 54–61.

Ferrero Camoletto, R. (2019) Questioning the sexy oldie: masculinity, age and sexuality in the Viagra era, in A. King, K. Almack and R.L. Jones (eds) *Intersections of Ageing, Gender and Sexualities: Multidisciplinary International Perspectives*, Policy Press, pp 209–22.

Ferrero Camoletto, R. (2021) Repairing sexual aging: Italian GPs' discourses in the Viagra era, in A. Jarrin and C. Pussetti (eds) *Remaking the Human: Cosmetic Technologies of Body Repair, Reshaping, and Replacement*, Berghahn, pp 53–74.

Ferrero Camoletto, R., Bertone, C. and Salis, F. (2015) Medicalizing male underperformance: expert discourses on male sexual health in Italy, *Salute e Societá*, 23: 183–205.

Ferrero Camoletto, R., Barrett, C. and Wentzell, E. (2020) Questioning the 'viagrization' of (hetero)sexual ageing, in, Z. Davy, A.C. Santos, C. Bertone, R. Thoreson and S.E. Wieringa (eds) *The SAGE Handbook of Global Sexualities*, Sage Publications Ltd.

Fishman, J. (2010) The making of Viagra: the biomedicalization of sexual dysfunction, in A.E. Clarke, L. Mamo, J.R. Fosket, J.R. Fishman and J.K. Shim (eds) *Biomedicalization: Technoscience, Health, and Illness in the US*, Duke University Press, pp 289–306.

Fletcher, P. (1972) The truth about impotence, in *Encyclopedia of Love and Sex*, Crescent Books, pp 163–5.

Fugh-Berman, A. (2015) The science of marketing: how pharmaceutical companies manipulated medical discourse on menopause, *Women's Reproductive Health*, 2(1): 18–23.

Goldstein, I. and Berman, J. (1998) Vasculogenic female sexual dysfunction: vaginal engorgement and clitoral erectile insufficiency syndromes, *International Journal of Impotence Research*, 10(Suppl.2): S84–90.

Goldstein, I. and Goldstein, S.W. (2024) Fighting for sexual medicine, *Sexual Medicine Reviews*, 12(2): 114–15.

Goldstein, S.W., Goldstein, I., Spana, C., Jordan, R. and Wills, S.T. (2023) Real-world use of bremelanotide in one sexual medicine clinic treating women with hypoactive sexual desire disorder, *The Journal of Sexual Medicine*, 20(Suppl.2).

Gott, M. (2005) *Sexuality, Sexual Health and Ageing*, Open University Press.

Gullette, M.M. (2003) What to do when being aged by culture: hidden narratives from the twentieth-century hormone debacle, *Generations*, 27(3): 71–6.

Gupta, K. (2019) *Medical Entanglements: Rethinking Feminist Debates About Healthcare*, Rutgers University Press.

Hitt, J. (2000) The second sexual revolution, *The New York Times Magazine*, 20 February, pp 34–41, 50, 62, 64, 68–9.

Illich, I. (1976) *Medical Nemesis: The Expropriation of Health*, Random House.

Islam, R.M., Bell, R.J., Green, S., Page, M.J. and Davis, S.R. (2019) Safety and efficacy of testosterone for women: a systematic review and meta-analysis of randomised controlled trial data, *The Lancet Diabetes & Endocrinology,* 7(10): 754–66.

Jarow, J., Kloner, R.A. and Holmes, A.M. (1998) *Viagra: How the Miracle Drug Happened and What It Can Do for You!* M. Evans and Co.

Johnson, E., Sjogren, E. and Asberg, C. (2011) Prescribing for the 'Swedish Viagra Man', *Clinical Pharmacology and Therapeutics*, 89(1): 15–16.

Johnson, L.A. (2017) Viagra goes generic: Pfizer to launch own little white pill, Washington Post [online] 6 December, Available from: https://www.washingtonpost.com/national/health-science/viagra-goes-generic-pfizer-to-launch-own-little-white-pill/2017/12/06/41f0e18a-daa7-11e7-a241-0848315642d0_story.html

Jutel, A. (2011) *Putting a Name to It: Diagnosis in Contemporary Society*, Johns Hopkins.

Jutel, A. and Mintzes, B. (2018) Female sexual dysfunction: medicalising desire, in B.M.Z. Cohen (ed) *Routledge International Handbook of Critical Mental Health*, Routledge, pp 162–8.

Katz, S. (2011) Hold on! Falling, embodiment and the materiality of old age, in M.J. Casper and P. Currah (eds) *Corpus: An Interdisciplinary Reader on Bodies and Knowledge*, Palgrave Macmillan, pp 187–206.

Kim, M.-J. and Uhl, K. (2011) Sex and lifestyle drugs: the pursuit of the fountain of youth, *Clinical Pharmacology and Therapeutics*, 89(1): 3–9.

Layton, J.B., Kim, Y., Alexander C., et al (2017) Association between direct-to-consumer advertising and testosterone testing and initiation in the United States, 2009–2013, *JAMA*, 317(11): 1159–66.

Loe, M. (2004a) *The Rise of Viagra: How the Little Blue Pill Changed Sex in America*, NYU Press.

Loe, M. (2004b) Sex and the senior woman: pleasure and danger in the Viagra era. *Sexualities*, 7(3): 303–26.

Loeb, C.A., Pardini-Furtado, T., Lavold, A., Bash, J.C., Mills, J.N. and Rajfer, J. (2024) A 25-year celebration of the little blue pill that revolutionized an industry, *Journal of Urology*, 211(5S).

Lowenstein, L., Shechter, A., Porst, H., Tripodi, F. and Reisman, Y. (2016) Physicians' attitudes towards androgen replacement therapy for male and female sexual dysfunction, *International Journal Of Impotence Research*, 28: 57.

Mamo, L. and Fishman, J. (2001) Potency in all the right places: Viagra as a technology of the gendered body, *Body and Society*, 7(4): 13–35.

Marshall, B.L. (2002) 'Hard science': gendered constructions of sexual dysfunction in the 'Viagra age', *Sexualities*, 5(2): 131–58.

Marshall, B.L. (2010) 'The nature of the body': anatomizing heterogender in sexual medicine, *Resources for Feminist Research*, 33(3–4): 17.

Marshall, B.L. and Katz, S. (2006) From androgyny to androgens: re-sexing the aging body, in, T. Calasanti and K. Slevin (eds) *Age Matters*, Routledge, pp 75–98.

Marshall, B.L. and Katz, S. (2012) The embodied life course: post-agesim or the re-naturalization of gender? *Societies*, 2: 222–34.

Marshall, B.L. (2020) 'Men are not women': biomedicine and the heterosexing of ageing bodies, in S. Pickard and J. Robinson (eds) *Ageing, the Body and the Gender Regime: Health, Illnes and Disease Across the Life Course*, Routledge, pp 128–42.

McKinlay, J.B. and Feldman, H.A. (1994) Age-related variation in sexual activity and interest in normal men: results from the Massachusetts male aging study, in A.S. Rossi (ed) *Sexuality Across the Life Course*, University of Chicago Press, pp 261–85.

Melchiode, G. and Sloan, B. (1999) *Beyond Viagra: A Commonsense Guide to Building a Healthy Sexual Relationship for Both Men and Women*, Owl Books (Henry Holt and Co.).

Morales, A. (1998) Preface, in A. Morales (ed) *Erectile Dysfunction: Issues in Current Pharmacotherapy*, Martin Dunitz Ltd, pp xv–vi.

Morales, A. (2008) The onset of late life hypogonadism, *The Aging Male*, 11(1): 43.

Morley, J.E. (2007) The politics of testosterone, *Journal of Sexual Medicine*, 4(3): 554–7.

National Institute of Health (1992) *NIH Consensus Statement: Impotence*, National Institute of Health.

Nieschlag, E., Swerdloff, R.S., Behre, H., Gooren, L.J., Kaufman, J.M., Legros, J.-J., Lunenfeld, B., Morley, J.E., Schulman, C., Wang, C., Wiedner, W. and Wu, F.C.W. (2005) Investigation, treatment and monitoring of late-onset hypogonadism in males, *The Aging Male*, 8(2): 56–8.

Oudshoorn, N. (1994) *Beyond the Natural Body: Towards an Archaeology of Sex Hormones*, Routledge.

Oxford English Dictionary (2001) *New Words List 2001* [online], Available from: https://public.oed.com/updates/new-words-list-september-2001/.

Portman, D.J., Brown, L., Yuan, J., Kissling, R. and Kingsberg, S.A. (2017) Flibanserin in postmenopausal women with hypoactive sexual desire disorder: results of the Plumeria study, *The Journal of Sexual Medicine*, 14(6): 834–42.

Potts, A. (2005) Cyborg masculinity in the Viagra era, *Sexualities, Evolution & Gender*, 7(1): 3–16.

Potts, A., Gavey, N., Grace, V. and Vares, T. (2003) The downside of Viagra: women's experiences and concerns, *Sociology of Health and Illness*, 25(7): 697–719.

Quartz staff (2018) After 20 years, Viagra has impacted so much more than just sex, *Quartz Magazine* [online], Available from: https://qz.com/quartzy/1238783/its-the-20th-anniversary-of-viagra-heres-how-its-changed-the-world

Roberts, C. (2002) 'A matter of embodied fact': sex hormones and the history of bodies, *Feminist Theory*, 3(1): 7–26.

Robinson, W.J. (1930) *A Practical Treatise on the Causes, Symptoms and Treatment of Sexual Impotence and Other Sexual Disorders in Men and Women* (15th edn), Critic and Guide Co.

Rohden, F. (2017) Male sexuality, medicalization and public health in Brazil, *Reproductive System and Sexual Disorder International Journal*, 1(2): 1–4.

Rohden, F. (2019) Adjusting hormones and constructing desires: new materialisations of female sexuality in Brazil, *Culture, Health & Sexuality*, 21(9): 1045–58.

Sengoopta, C. (2001) Transforming the testicle: science, medicine and masculinity, 1800–1951, *Medicina nei Secoli*, 13(3): 637–55.

Sengoopta, C. (2006) *The Most Secret Quintessence of Life: Sex, Glands and Hormones, 1850–1950*, University of Chicago Press.

Spielmans, G.I. and Ellefson, E.M. (2024) Small effects, questionable outcomes: bremelanotide for hypoactive sexual desire disorder, *The Journal of Sex Research*, 61(4): 540–61.

Squier, S. (1999) Incubabies and rejuvenates: the traffic between technologies of reproduction and age-extension, in K. Woodward (ed) *Figuring Age: Women, Bodies, Generation*, Indiana University Press, pp 88–111.

Stock, W. and Moser, C. (2001) Feminist sex therapy in the age of Viagra, in P.J. Kleinplatz (ed) *New Directions in Sex Therapy*, Brunner-Routledge, pp 139–62.

Tetley, J., Lee, D.M., Nazroo, J. and Hinchliff, S. (2018) Let's talk about sex – what do older men and women say about their sexual relations and sexual activities? A qualitative analysis of Elsa Wave 6 data, *Ageing and Society*, 38(3): 497–521.

Thangaraju, P., Velmurugan, H. and Ty, S.S. (2022) Drug flibanserin – in hypoactive sexual desire disorder, *Gynecology and Obstetrics Clinical Medicine*, 2(2): 91–5.

Tiefer, L. (2006) The Viagra phenomenon, *Sexualities*, 9(3): 273–94.

Vares, T., Potts, A., Gavey, N. and Grace, V. (2007) Reconceptualizing cultural narratives of mature women's sexuality in the Viagra era, *Journal of Aging Studies*, 21(2): 153–64.

Vaughn, S.C. (1998) *Viagra: A Guide to the Phenomenal Potency-Promoting Drug*, Pocket Books (Simon and Schuster).

Wallach, I., Beauchamp, J., Alarie, M. and Miller, G. (2020) Between exploration, pleasure, and performance: sexual enhancement medication use among older gay and heterosexual men, *The Journal of Sex Research*, 57(8): 1–9.

Wang, C., Nieschlag, E., Swerdloff, R.S., Behre, H., Hellstrom, W.J., Gooren, L.J., Kaufman, J.M., Legros, J.-J., Lunenfeld, B., Morales, A., Morley, J.E., Schulman, C., Thompson, I.M., Weidner, W. and Wu, F.C.W. (2008) ISA, ISSAM, EAU, EAA and ASA recommendations: investigation, treatment and monitoring of late-onset hypogonadism in males, *The Aging Male*, 12(1): 5–12.

Watkins, E.S. (2008) Medicine, masculinity and the disappearance of the male menopause in the 1950s, *Social History of Medicine*, 21(2): 329–44.

Wentzell, E. (2011) Marketing silence, public health stigma and the discourse of risky gay Viagra use in the US, *Body & Society*, 17(4): 105–25.

Wentzell, E. (2013) *Maturing Masculinities: Aging, Chronic Illness and Viagra in Mexico*, Duke University Press.

Wentzell, E. (2017) Erectile dysfunction as successful aging in Mexico, in S. Lamb (ed) *Successful Aging as a Contemporary Obsession: Global Perspectives*, Rutgers University Press.

Wentzell, E. (2021) Time and collective biology: relationships between individual and societal life course ideologies in Mexican men's sexual health treatment, *Anthropology & Aging*, 42(1): 66–88.

Wentzell, E. and Labuski, C. (2020) Role of medical anthropology in understanding cultural differences in sexuality, in D.L. Rowland and E.A. Jannini (eds) *Cultural Differences and the Practices of Sexual Medicine: A Guide for Sexual Health Practitioners*, Springer International, pp 23–35.

Werland, R. (2004) Manhood checkup, *Chicago Tribune*, 27 June, p 9.

Whitehead, E.D. and Malloy, T. (1999) *Viagra: The Wonder Drug for Peak Performance*, Dell Books.

Wilson, R.A. (1966) *Feminine Forever*, Evans.

Wyllie, M. (2003) Adam and the andropause, *British Journal of Urology International*, 91: 883–4.

Wyllie, M. (2005) The hunt for pink Viagra, *British Journal of Urology International*, 95(1): 181–2.

7

The sexuality of older persons in the digital world

Liat Ayalon and Ateret Gewirtz-Meydan

This chapter addresses two major changes that have taken place in the past few decades: the demographic shift, which has resulted in a growing number of older persons and in the ageing of societies worldwide; and the digital revolution, which is reconstructing all spheres of life including older age, ageing and sexuality. The chapter seeks to expand the understanding of the intersection between digital media and sexuality in later life. This intersection will be reviewed in relation to research questions: (1) how digital media represents the sexuality of older persons; and (2) how older persons use digital media for love and sex.

These two questions possibly represent an emerging transition from desexualisation of older persons as asexual, inadequate, unfit and lacking desire for sex and sexuality in traditional media and discourse to the resexualisation of older age and ageing in digital media as agents who are capable of choosing, experimenting, and benefiting from online sexual opportunities and innovations. Gender, age, sex and sexuality are not only biological, but have strong social influences and contexts (Heaphy, 2007). Some commentators view digital media as a particularly egalitarian mechanism that can sidestep discrimination based on physical appearance, gender or age, and allow older persons agency beyond societal constraints. Moreover, digital media allows for the expression of various sexual desires and preferences that might not be easily shared in public otherwise (Adams et al, 2003), and thus it can be viewed as a liberating sexual tool. However, despite the promise of digital media, we also highlight barriers to inclusion and representation of older persons in digital media as well as negative and often unintended consequences of digital media use for sexual purposes.

Throughout the chapter, we highlight the intersection of age with gender, given the understanding that we all possess more than a single attribute of relevance. In the case of sexuality, there is no doubt that gender plays a major role not only in desexualisation of older persons, but also in opportunities for resexualisation. Although this is only briefly discussed, we also highlight other attributes of relevance such as level of education, socioeconomic status, physical ability and sexual orientation. The intersections of age with other forms of difference reflect the understanding that the whole is greater than the sum of its parts.

The representation of older persons in media

This section discusses how digital media portrays or reconstructs sexuality in later life. The illustration of later life sexuality in digital media may shape societal views on the sexuality of older persons but, also, and maybe most importantly, shape what older persons think about their own sexuality, through the internalisation of messages conveyed by digital media. The representation of older persons in media, including digital media, has changed over time and is largely context-dependent and thus affected both by the country and its sociocultural characteristics as well as by the historical period (Loos and Ivan, 2018). Representations are also medium-dependent and differ across formal mechanisms of communication, such as newspapers or television, and informal mechanisms, such as online social networks, including X (formerly Twitter), Instagram or Facebook (Rajendran and Thesinghraja, 2014). As this chapter attends to digital media and older persons' sexuality, our focus is primarily on the latter forms of communication, which tend to be less formal and thus, may reflect somewhat less censored messages and attitudes.

Although the chapter is focused on older persons' sexuality, it is important to acknowledge the fact that stigma and stereotypes concerning older persons' sexuality online do not occur in a vacuum, but rather are influenced by the general social context. Hence, we will start by reviewing the general stereotypes of older persons and old age, followed by stereotypes of older persons and technology use as they may relate to older persons' sexual online representation. We will then conclude by discussing older persons' sexuality as depicted by online media.

We argue that stereotypes of older persons' sexuality represent one form of ageism, which is known as a bias in the way we think, feel or act towards people because of their age (Ayalon and Tesch-Römer, 2018; Simpson et al, 2018). Although ageism can be both positive and negative, and can be directed towards adults of any age group, our focus in this chapter is on negative ageist stereotypes towards older persons. According to Fiske (2018), stereotypes of different minority groups can be classified along two axes of warmth and competence. Different minority groups are judged along these two categories, with older persons being seen as high on warmth, but low on competence (Cuddy et al, 2005). These same stereotypes also are reflected in media representations. For instance, during the current pandemic, older persons were portrayed as a burden to society, given the fact that they made more demands on healthcare systems and used scarce resources, supposedly at the expense of the younger generations (Meisner, 2021). At the same time, there were also heroic stories about older persons sacrificing their lives for the sake of others, thus the goodness and kindness of older persons were emphasised along the 'warmth' quality (Allen et al, 2021).

Ageism, however, does not occur out of context, but often in interaction between chronological age and other socio-cultural characteristics, such as gender, race/ethnicity, or socioeconomic status (Krekula et al, 2018). Clearly, the ageing experiences of poor Black older women are not comparable to that of rich white older men. Hence, both societal stereotypes of these individuals and their own self-perceptions of ageing are likely to be impacted not only by their chronological age, but also by their various attributes.

The representation of older persons in media, including online digital media

Older persons increasingly consume their health information, including sexual education from online sources (Minichiello et al, 2013; Fileborn et al, 2017). As such, it is important to consider challenges faced by this population when exposed to online information. Specifically, research has shown that older persons are more likely to accept fake information as real (Brashier and Schacter, 2020). Hence, they might be particularly vulnerable to disinformation about their sexual health. This challenge might be further enhanced by the limited sexual education provided to older persons throughout their lives (May, 2006). Thus, older persons might be lacking the tools to judge the adequacy of online sexual information. As older persons are notoriously known for spreading and sharing information online more so than younger generations, exposure to fake or inaccurate information might be particularly problematic in their case (Ayalon, 2024).

Over the years, both the content and the frequency of older persons' representations in the media have changed. The initial media representation of older persons was highly negative, emphasising undesired qualities and vulnerabilities associated with older age. Over time, however, older persons' representation has become overly positive, portraying old age as a continuation of middle age and advocating for a successful ageing model (Loos and Ivan, 2018). Consistently, older persons' presence in media including digital media has increased over time (Lee et al, 2007). Chivers (2019) has termed the phrase 'silvering screen' to describe the increasing presence of older protagonists in the movies. This has been attributed to the increasing presence of the baby boom generation, the target audience of this line of movies.

The intersection between age and gender in media representations is highly pronounced. In the case of women, researchers have argued that their representations have gone through four stages. The first stage involves the complete invisibility of older women. The second stage concerns the use of very clear and ageist stereotypes to represent older women, during which, and regardless of the presentation of older women, their sexuality has been silenced. The third stage represents the ghettoisation of older women in the media by creating shows that feature solely older women. The fourth stage should represent the integration of women in mainstream media (Lemish and Muhlbauer, 2012). A similar transition was also used to describe the representation of lesbian, gay, bisexual, transgender, queer and intersex (LGBTQ&I) older persons, who have transitioned from being invisible and not present at all in the media to being depicted as victims and more recently as icons and extraordinary symbols of resilience (Hurd et al, 2020). In contrast to women and people of less traditional sexual pathways, men, who represent the hegemonic social group, continue to capture leading roles as protagonists even in old age.

Media portrayal of older persons and technology use

When it comes to technology use and older persons' representation, the stereotype of incompetence is particularly pronounced (Mariano et al, 2021). Older persons are thought to demonstrate a low mastery of technology and digital media and both advertisements and media reports highlight these shortcomings of older persons. Consistently, the prevailing stereotype of older persons and technology stresses their inadequate ability to use or lack of interest in using new technologies (Wandke et al, 2012). As such, the entire representation of older persons, including older persons' sexuality in digital media, is coloured by this frame.

It is not only the stereotypes of older persons and technology use, which are negative, but online discourse as well tends to be ageist, stressing older persons' vulnerabilities and incompetence (Xu, 2021). Moreover, the one study that has looked at online social groups on Facebook has found that the portrayal of older persons has been quite negative. Even designated online Facebook groups which specifically target older persons, highlight their shortcomings (Levy et al, 2014). Hence, when it comes to older persons' representations within digital media, the negative portrayal of older persons also concerns their technological challenges to master it.

Media portrayal of older persons' sexuality

The sexual stereotypes of older persons concern the views of older persons as asexual and unattractive (Walz, 2002; Kenny, 2013). However, whereas men are generally viewed as competent and attractive even in old age, women tend to lose their socio-sexual appeal in middle age. This distinction is explained by evolutionary theories (Buss, 1989). Specifically, women are thought to lose their attractiveness given their inability to reproduce, which begins in middle age. Men, on the other hand, can reproduce for a longer period, and thus, their sex appeal diminishes later in life. Moreover, whereas women are judged by their looks (Kenalemang, 2021), men are more likely to be judged by their financial status and career achievements. Consistently, a recent study has concluded that although both men and women are largely invisible in media, women's invisibility is particularly pronounced (Edström, 2018).

One way to learn about the sexual portrayal of men and women is through the examination of dating sites. These sites tend to portray older age as a continuation of middle age (Gewirtz-Meydan and Ayalon, 2018). Both men and women are visually presented with limited or no wrinkles. Women are usually shown with coloured hair, whereas men may have grey hair, but still physically fit and no wrinkles (Gewirtz-Meydan and Ayalon, 2018). The terms used to describe older persons also tend to be problematic. Even websites directly geared to cater to the preferences of older persons use neutralising terms such as 'mature' or 'senior', possibly attempting to downplay age and disguise the target age group of older persons. Related to this, the terms used to describe women are often humiliating, though somewhat ambivalent at times, emphasising negative or inappropriate qualities such as 'the cougar', which may reflect some sneaking admiration in addition to negative judgement. In contrast, based on data derived from the same online dating sites, men, were not portrayed using such negative terms (Ayalon and Gewirtz-Meydan, 2017). This, again, demonstrates the intersection between ageism and sexism where women are the target of substantially more negative stereotypes (Roy and Ayalon, 2020). Within this context it is also important to note that dating sites present mainly heterosexual relations, thus, advocating for a heteronormative perspective of older persons' sexuality (Gewirtz-Meydan and Ayalon, 2018).

The sexual representation of older persons is also highly influenced by the pharmaceutical industry. Specifically, the appearance of Viagra in the 1990s was portrayed as a lifechanging invention that completely transformed older persons' sexuality (Ayalon and Gewirtz-Meydan, 2019). The pharmaceutical industry has portrayed male inability to perform as a problem, a physiological dysfunction that must be overcome using medication. This clearly ignores the fact that human sexuality is highly influenced by social and psychological factors as well (Marshall, 2008). Although many physicians tend to see this portrayal as advantageous and are pleased with the involvement of the pharmaceutical companies in older persons' sexual education, it possibly has negative implications for older persons, who might view pharmaceutical sexual treatments as a cure-all (Ayalon and Gewirtz-Meydan, 2019).

Likewise, women's sexuality has become increasingly more medicalised over time. Women's sexual problems are largely grouped under the umbrella term, female sexual dysfunction (Hartley, 2006). As with older men, women's sexuality and changes in sexuality are mainly accounted for by hormonal and biological changes, and psychological or social circumstances receive less attention. The medicalisation of women's sexuality also creates clear messages about the way women's sexuality should be and how deviations from the norm should be treated by medication.

For instance, hormone replacement therapy (HRT) has shaped women's views of sexuality and of femininity (Whittaker, 1998) by reconstructing the view of ageing women as unnatural. Reportedly, menopause has been reconstructed by the pharmaceutical industry as representing a deficiency, requiring pharmaceutical interventions (Burrell, 2009). This reconstruction of natural processes as representing pathology can compromise women's health and well-being. For instance, a qualitative study of 30 American women has shown that they were indifferent to possible risks associated with taking HRT for a prolonged period. This indifference was explained by the belief in the power of HRT to preserve youth and prevent diseases (Hunter et al, 2020).

Reconstructing ageing in line with the pharmaceutical agenda enhances the association of sexual performance with the successful ageing model. This model portrays older age as a continuation of middle age. Older persons are expected to perform cognitively, mentally, and socially as they performed when they were younger (Calasanti, 2015). A major problem with the successful ageing model is that it does not adequately reflect reality. Specifically, research has shown that only 8.5 per cent of all older Europeans over the age of 65 (Hank, 2011) and as many as 11.9 per cent of older Americans can be classified as successful agers (McLaughlin et al, 2010). Consistently, only 38.9 per cent of men aged 75–85 are sexually active (Lindau and Gavrilova, 2010). Hence, being sexually active in old or very old age may not be the norm, yet, it is portrayed as a 'curable' pathology by the pharmaceutical industry. Moreover, the ability to perform sexually is not only determined by biological and hormonal functioning, but also by the availability or lack of availability of a partner (DeLamater and Koepsel, 2015). Stressing the 'failure' of older men and women to perform further highlights their vulnerability and makes the distinction between successful and unsuccessful older persons even more pronounced, at times, at the expanse of older persons' physical and mental health.

What is the impact of negative online stereotypes of older persons' sexuality?

The stereotype embodiment theory suggests that people internalise negative stereotypes of older persons, age and ageing throughout their lives (Levy, 2009). Even at a very young age, people already hold certain stereotypes towards older persons. As they grow older, these stereotypes become evident and impactful. The problem is that holding negative self-stereotypes towards one's ageing self has shown to have a negative impact on older persons' health and well-being (Levy et al, 2002; Kotter-Grühn et al, 2009). Negative self-perceptions of ageing are associated with increased morbidity, greater functional disability, higher levels of depression and even increased mortality (Sargent-Cox et al, 2012, 2014; Han and Richardson, 2015).

When it comes to self-perceptions of one's sexuality, it is likely that men and women internalise different stereotypes and perceive themselves as asexual, irrelevant and not appealing. Compared with men, women are exposed to substantially more negative sexual stereotypes at a younger age (Hinchliff and Gott, 2008). This could potentially explain the preference of men to date younger women (Alterovitz and Mendelsohn, 2009). This may also explain the reliance and interest of women in the beauty and anti-ageing industries in an attempt to conceal visible signs of ageing (Clarke and Griffin, 2008).

The representation of older persons as asexual also carries negative implications. Specifically, if older persons do not think of themselves as sexual beings, they are less likely to rely on protected sex, for instance (Kenny, 2013). This, in turn, may result in higher infection rates in this population of older persons. Indeed, research has shown that the rates of sexually-transmitted diseases are particularly pronounced in this population group of older persons (Bodley-Tickell et al, 2008). This group likely received limited sexual education when young and currently has fewer opportunities to learn about sexuality and sexual risk behaviors compared with younger generations (Ayalon et al, 2019).

Stereotype threat occurs when individuals are at risk of confirming negative stereotypes about their social group (Lamont et al, 2015). Under such circumstances, individuals perform more poorly, especially when the situation evokes a threat to their group identity. In the case of older persons, stereotype threat has shown to be particularly detrimental to their cognitive functioning (Barber and Mather, 2014). When it comes to sexual functioning, given the prominence of advertisements concerning pharmaceutical enhancers to sexual dysfunction, particularly men, are likely affected by advertisements that portray their sexual performance as inadequate without artificial enhancers. Hence, beliefs about dysfunctional sexual performance are likely to act as a self-fulfilling prophecy.

In sum, this section reviewed the portrayal of older persons over traditional and digital media. We started by reflecting on the representation (and often lack of representation) of older persons over traditional and digital media and then transitioned to reviewing common stereotypes and beliefs about older persons' limited or inadequate ability to use technology and digital media. Subsequently, we discussed the representation of older persons' sex and sexuality, which concerns only one aspect of their social media portrayal. Overall, despite differences between men and women, we conclude that to the most part, older persons' sexuality is silenced both offline and online. Moreover, normal sexual changes associated with ageing are portrayed as pathological and requiring medical interventions. This aims to establish older age as a continuation of middle age. Under such circumstances, for the most part, digital media does not fulfil the egalitarian promise of liberating older persons from the ties of societal stereotypes and norms, but rather enhances existing stereotypes and norms of older persons as asexual beings and portrays natural sexual processes as aberrant. Moreover, although the portrayal of older men and women differs, both older men and older women are exposed to negative stereotypes, which silence their sexuality.

The use of digital media for sex and love in later life

Although older persons consistently have lower rates of technology adoption than the general public, reports indicate older persons are embracing technology at a rapid pace (Pew Research Center, 2017). For example, based on a non-partisan US think tank, over a period of 5 years, the number of older persons using a smartphone has doubled. Internet use among seniors has also risen steadily over the last decade and a half. In early 2000, just 14 per cent of older persons were using the internet; more than a decade later, 67 per cent of adults aged 65 and older say they use the internet. Finally, digital media use among older persons is also steadily increasing, with 34 per cent of Americans aged 65 and up reporting using social networking sites such as Facebook or X (Pew Research Center, 2017).

According to the Pew Research Center (2017), older persons use the media as a platform to consume news, seek information, share experiences and connect with friends and family. Limited information is available on whether and how older persons use digital media for love and sex purposes. A recent study examining online sexual activities among older persons has categorised these in three ways (Scandurra et al, 2022): non-arousal activities (such as visiting sexual educational websites or chatting on dating websites), solitary arousal activities (watching pornography), and partnered arousal activities, which require the participation of at least one other individual (such as engaging in webcam sex or sexual chat, activities requiring virtual interactive participation of at least two people). Another study conducted among 3,816 European older persons found that older persons use digital media for three main purposes regarding sex and love: seeking a partner, sexual self enhancement and seeking information or advice. It is important to note that twice as many men as women were likely to use digital media for these purposes, with the most common online use being pornography consumption (Træen et al, 2018).

Using digital media for seeking a partner (committed or casual)

Many older persons maintain interest in intimate partner relationships and actively seek partners online (Malta, 2007). Online dating websites are gaining popularity as a convenient way to connect with potential partners. A growing number of older persons are using online dating sites and 'apps' to meet new people (Wada et al, 2015). In 2019, 19 per cent of people aged 55–64 reported having tried dating apps along with 13 per cent of older persons aged 64 and above (Pew Research Center, 2020).

The American Association of Retired Persons (AARP, 2013) conducted a survey to understand the reasons why older persons use online dating sites. According to the survey, older persons think they can meet a broader range of people (23 per cent) through online sites; they do not have to reply or talk to people they do not want to (20 per cent); and because a friend recommended it (14 per cent). Regarding what older persons are seeking, 48 per cent report using online dating sites to find a serious relationship, 26 per cent wish to find friendship and companionship, and only 14 per cent seek casual dating. The AARP survey aligns with a study conducted among older persons in Australia (Malta, 2007). According to the latter study, relationships that have begun online were for the most part meaningful, intimate and long-lasting. A small proportion of older persons also enjoyed flirting online with others and some were involved in extra-dyadic relationships, which represent a breach or infidelity of agreed upon monogamic, dyadic relationships.

Scarce data on the prevalence of older men and women using digital media to seek partners make it impossible to determine gender differences in use of digital media for sexual, erotic or love-related purposes. It can be assumed that participation in online dating in later life follows the overall trend of gender differences in online dating participation, in which men are significantly more likely than women to participate in online dating (Abramova et al, 2016).

Studies provide insight into gender differences in what older men and women might want from online dating. According to a recent study, older women sought a partner who was honest and would share leisure activities with them, while older men sought women who were physically attractive and would provide emotional support (Watson and Stelle, 2021). An analysis of 600 internet personal adverts posted on online dating sites, revealed that, with age, men desired women increasingly younger than themselves, whereas women desired older men until ages 75 and over, when they sought men younger than themselves. The authors concluded that in line with evolutionary theory, men were more likely to seek physical attractiveness, attributed to younger women, but women were more likely to value prestige and power, offered by older men (Alterovitz and Mendelsohn, 2009).

Using digital media for sexual self enhancement

Digital media is becoming a medium through which sexuality is expressed. However, due to limited research in this area, it may be impossible to determine the exact number of older persons who are using digital media for sexual expression and stimulation (Adams et al, 2003). It is assumed that older persons underreport their use of digital media for sexual self-enhancement because of the threat of stigma if they acknowledge that they are not only sexual but that they engage in (historically) unconventional means of expressing it (Adams et al, 2003).

Sexual self-enhancement can come in two main forms: solitary (such as watching pornography), and partnered (for example, engaging in webcam sex or sexual chat, activities which require a virtual interactive participation of at least two people). Research on the engagement of older persons in both forms of activity is scarce. Yet a recent study indicates that using digital media for sexual self enhancement is popular among older persons, with a total of 58.1 per cent of older Italians reporting using the internet for sexual self-enhancement at least two to three times during the previous month (Scandurra et al, 2022).

Individuals who masturbate frequently may have a higher sex drive or place a higher value on their sex life, which motivates them to watch pornography and get pleasure out of it, as sex is more important to them. Considering solitary sexual activities, pornography use is one of the most common forms. Overall, the use of the internet to watch pornography decreases with increasing age (Price et al, 2016; Træen et al, 2018; Scandurra et al, 2022), yet using the internet to read or watch erotica or pornography is still one of the most common activities connected to sex and love in which older men and women engage, though men are substantially more likely to admit to the use of digital media for this purpose (Træen et al, 2018). The decrease of pornography use with age can reflect both the decrease in sexual interest and activity with increasing age (Træen et al, 2017), as well as a general lower internet use in older age groups (Ayalon et al, 2019). In a study conducted among 3,816 European older persons, pornography use was associated with a higher frequency of masturbation only in men (Træen et al, 2018), while in another study conducted among 799 Czech older persons, pornography use was associated with a higher frequency of masturbation in both men and women (Sevcikova et al, 2021).

The partnered online sexual activities of older persons are much less studied. Thus, it is hard to determine how widespread these practices are. Although there has been little research in this area, it appears that older persons are pursuing cyber-sex and enjoying it as part of their sexual repertoire (Malta, 2007). According to a study among 114 older persons aged 52–79 years old, partnered online sexual activities were the least common form of online sexual activities compared with other forms such as pornography use and using online dating apps (Scandurra et al, 2022). However, partnered online sexual activities were still reported by one out of three older persons in the study (Scandurra et al, 2022). Interestingly, Scandurra et al (2022) pointed out that engaging in solitary sexual activities online (in comparison to partnered online sexual activities) is more common among non-heterosexual older persons. This may reflect the intersection between ageism and heterosexism, which places LGBTQI older persons in a more vulnerable and lonelier place and forces them to return to the 'closet' in later life (Hafford-Letchfield, 2008). As such, expressing their sexuality on an anonymous digital media can be valuable for sexual health but may also reinforce the stigma on LGBTQI older persons and drive them even further into the 'closet'.

Finally in this section, while not categorised as solitary or partnered, another main use of the internet for sexual self-enhancement concerns visiting online sex shops and buying sex products. Online sex shops offer sex toys, vibrators, erotic books, videos and clothing but also medication and natural supplements that are toted as capable of raising a person's libido and increasing erectile strength and vaginal lubrication. These products are offered to all customers but are often advertised and tailored specifically for older populations (Adams et al, 2003). The anonymous and immediate purchase of such products frees older persons from the stigma they might face concerning later life sexuality and from the fear of purchasing from local vendors face-to-face (Adams et al, 2003).

Indeed, a study conducted among older persons based in four different European countries found that buying sex products is common (Træen et al, 2018). In the study, both men and women who masturbated more were more likely to use the internet to buy sex products than individuals who did not masturbate (Træen et al, 2018). In a study conducted among 799 internet-recruited Czechs aged 50–96, visiting sex shops was more frequent among men (Sevcikova et al, 2021). Higher odds of visiting online sex shops were associated with masturbation and greater importance for sex in both men and women (Sevcikova et al, 2021).

Using media for seeking information and advice about sex

Media (including traditional forms such as television and magazines) and the internet are two of the most preferred sources of information to learn about sex in later life, with the internet being the most common source used (Fileborn et al, 2017). Older persons use the internet to source a wide range of information on topics such as sexual transmitted diseases and safer sex, sexual dysfunction and ageing and sexuality and sexual pleasure (Fileborn et al, 2017). Older persons also satisfy their needs for information, advice and support on sexual matters with sex-related discussions in older persons' online communities (Berdychevsky and Nimrod, 2015). These communities are popular and much needed given the reality of limited alternatives for open and direct sex-related communication in later life. These online communities offer notable potential for helping people to cope with the three primary sexual vulnerabilities that occur in later life: health issues and life circumstances that affect sexuality; difficulties communicating with health care providers about sex-related problems; and limited access to sexual health information (Berdychevsky and Nimrod, 2015). As use of the internet increases among older persons, it is likely that this will be a key site for education, and a space in which specific resources for older persons should be made available.

A population-based survey among older persons has shown that 15 per cent of men and women who experience sexual difficulties will use the internet or other forms of media to seek help (Laumann et al, 2009). According to a recent study, ascribing importance to sex, feeling dissatisfied with the frequency of sex and struggling with erectile difficulties (for men) were predictors of seeking sexual-related information online (Sevcikova et al, 2021).

Hinchliff and Gott (2011) highlight the advantages of using the internet for seeking information on sex in later life: the internet allows access to a substantial body of literature on sexual health and sexuality aimed directly at older persons and also facilitates greater access to sex aids in a way that overcomes the barriers of geographic location and physical ability. The internet also provides anonymity, which can be extremely important in older age when experiencing sexual ageism and the stigma of being asexual (Gewirtz-Meydan et al, 2018; Simpson et al, 2018). Although using the internet to seek information on sex has great advantages, older persons are also aware of the risks and pitfalls of seeking information online and describe themselves as critical of internet material (Fileborn et al, 2017). Older persons who use the internet to seek information about sex are selective about which sites they use and look for certain criteria in judging the quality of information provided. Reportedly, academic information provided by universities or medical institutes, or information provided by governments was more likely to be judged as trustworthy (Fileborn et al, 2017).

It is clear, then, that digital media have become a means through which sexuality is expressed and shaped. Concurrently, older persons are increasingly using digital media creatively to enhance their sexuality and sexual experiences. There are too many unknowns to provide a reliable summary of how often older persons use digital media for sex and love purposes and in what ways. However, the literature reviewed on this matter suggests that older persons use digital media for many of the same reasons as their younger counterparts, as well as for unique pursuits. The main uses of digital media for love and sex purposes in later life are to seek a partner (committed or casual), for sexual self enhancement (solitary or partnered), to buy sex products and visit online sex shops and to seek information and advice about sex. Without doubt, sexual expression on the internet has facilitative potential for older persons. It allows older persons to express their sexuality, partner with people and get help and advice regarding their sexuality.

From desexualisation to resexualisation of older men and women via digital technology

This chapter has highlighted the important role that traditional and more recently digital media play in older persons' sexuality. Digital media can serve as a place to develop a perspective on older persons' sexuality and as a place to seek sexual information, relations or stimuli. The chapter highlights the need to examine the relations between later life and digital media in both directions. Whereas digital media plays a central role in shaping and many times constraining views of sexuality in later life, it may also provide a platform for agency and liberty concerning older persons' sexual self-definition and action, which to some extent can be free of societal constraints.

Our review shows that digital media does not go without limitations and often fosters exposure to inaccurate, fake or biased information, which may foster stereotypical perceptions and expectations concerning one's body and sexual life throughout the life course and especially in older age. Moreover, ageist erotophobia likely colours not only real-life sexual relations and opportunities of older persons (Simpson et al, 2017), but also online activities. This finding is particularly disconcerting given the growing reliance of older persons and society at large on digital media. Moreover, as older persons are particularly susceptible to consuming and spreading fake news (Ayalon and Roy, 2023), which may be even more harmful for this growing segment of the population. Moreover, as digital media tends to have fewer checks and balances than traditional media sources, it is likely that future generations of older persons will be even more negatively impacted by online stereotypes and prejudices of older persons as asexual and of normal changes associated with ageing as pathological. This suggests that digital media may not represent an opportunity for freedom and equity, but rather strengthens the norms and constrains imposed by society via implicit and explicit online stereotypical messages. As the use of digital media has increased over time, it is important to ensure that older persons are exposed to accurate sexual information that does not discriminate them based on their age and/or sexual orientation and preferences.

On the other hand, via the presumed privacy, and richness of opportunities it offers, digital media also represents an opportunity to free older persons from the chains of societal stereotypical portrayal of them as asexual and of their sexuality as deviant or pathological. Instead, digital media allows older persons, even those with substantial physical impairments, to engage in varied sexual behaviors and to explore their sexuality in the presumed privacy and openness fostered by online media. However, it is important to acknowledge the fact that many times the opportunities to explore sex and sexuality online come at the expense of others. For instance, pornography, at least in its more traditional form, is notoriously known for strengthening hetero-patriarchal stereotypes and behaviours (Heredia, 2022).

Although promising, given the strong biases identified in the representations of older persons as asexual and pathological, it is unclear whether indeed digital media fulfils its promise. Further research is needed to better understand how the online portrayal of sex and sexuality of older persons impacts their sexual online activities. Moreover, there is still a dearth of information on the topic, especially from the perspective of the LGBTQI community, but also from the perspective of older persons in varied countries, outside North America, Australia or Europe. Further research will benefit from integrating the two pathways through which the encounter between older persons and digital media takes place in the context of sex and sexuality. In addition, although we briefly discussed intersectionality, with a particular attention to gender differences between men and women, there is a clear need for further exploration of intersectionality and its effects not only on older persons' sexual representations, but also on their ability and preferences to use digital media to enhance their sex life and sexuality.

References

American Association of Retired Persons (2013) AARP online dating survey [online], Available from: https://www.aarp.org/research/topics/life/info-2014/online-dating-sites-survey.html

Abramova, O., Baumann, A., Krasnova, H. and Buxmann, P. (2016) Gender differences in online dating: what do we know so far? A systematic literature review, *2016 49th Hawaii International Conference on System Sciences (HICSS)*, 3858–67.

Adams, M., Oye, J. and Parker, T. (2003) Sexuality of older adults and the internet: from sex education to cybersex, *Sexual and Relationship Therapy*, 18(3): 405–15.

Allen, L.D., Odziemczyk, I.Z., Perek-Białas, J. and Ayalon, L. (2021) We should be at the back of the line': a frame analysis of old age within the distribution order of the COVID vaccine, *The Gerontologist*, 61(8): 1317–25.

Alterovitz, S.S.-R. and Mendelsohn, G.A. (2009) Partner preferences across the life span: online dating by older adults, *Psychology and Aging*, 24(2): 513–17.

Ayalon, L. (2024) Age differences in the context of climate change: does exposure to a fake consensus statement make a difference?, *Plos One*, 19(3): e0298219.

Ayalon, L. and Gewirtz-Meydan, A. (2017) Senior, mature or single: a qualitative analysis of homepage advertisements of dating sites for older adults, *Computers in Human Behavior*, 75: 876–82.

Ayalon, L. and Tesch-Römer, C. (2018) *Contemporary Perspectives on Ageism*, Springer Nature.

Ayalon, L. and Gewirtz-Meydan, A. (2019) Physicians' moral dilemmas in the age of Viagra, *Men and Masculinities*, 24(4): 690–707.

Ayalon, L. and Roy, S. (2023) The role of chronological age in climate change attitudes, feelings, and behavioral intentions: the case of null results, *PloS One*, 18(6): e0286901.

Ayalon, L., Levkovich, I., Gewirtz-Meydan, A. and Karkabi, K. (2019) A life course perspective on the ways older men and women discuss sexual issues, *Archives of Sexual Behavior*, 48: 911–19.

Barber, S.J. and Mather, M. (2014) Stereotype threat in older adults: when and why does it occur and who is most affected?, in P. Verhaeghen and C. Hertzog (eds) *The Oxford Handbook of Emotion, Social Cognition and Problem Solving in Adulthood*, Oxford University Press, pp 302–19.

Berdychevsky, L. and Nimrod, G. (2015) 'Let's talk about sex': discussions in seniors' online communities, *Journal of Leisure Research*, 47(4): 467–84.

Bodley-Tickell, A.T., Olowokure, B., Bhaduri, S., White, D.J., Ward, D., Ross, J.D., Smith, G., Duggal, H.V. and Goold, P. (2008) Trends in sexually transmitted infections (other than HIV) in older people: analysis of data from an enhanced surveillance system, *Sexually Transmitted Infections*, 84(4): 312–17.

Brashier, N.M. and Schacter, D.L. (2020) Aging in an era of fake news, *Current Directions in Psychological Science*, 29(3): 316–23.

Burrell, B.A. (2009) The replacement of the replacement in menopause: hormone therapy, controversies, truth and risk, *Nursing Inquiry*, 16(3): 212–22.

Buss, D.M. (1989) Toward an evolutionary psychology of human mating, *Behavioral and Brain Sciences*, 12(1): 39–49.

Calasanti, T. (2015) Combating ageism: how successful is successful aging?, *The Gerontologist*, 56(6): 1093–101.

Chivers, S. (2019) *The Silvering Screen*, University of Toronto Press.

Clarke, L.H. and Griffin, M. (2008) Visible and invisible ageing: beauty work as a response to ageism, *Ageing & Society*, 28(5): 653–74.

Cuddy, A.J., Norton, M.I. and Fiske, S.T. (2005) This old stereotype: the pervasiveness and persistence of the elderly stereotype, *Journal of Social Issues*, 61(2): 267–85.

DeLamater, J. and Koepsel, E. (2015) Relationships and sexual expression in later life: a biopsychosocial perspective, *Sexual and Relationship Therapy*, 30(1): 37–59.

Edström, M. (2018) Visibility patterns of gendered ageism in the media buzz: a study of the representation of gender and age over three decades, *Feminist Media Studies*, 18(1): 77–93.

Fileborn, B., Lyons, A., Hinchliff, S., Brown, G., Heywood, W. and Minichiello, V. (2017) Learning about sex in later life: sources of education and older Australian adults, *Sex Education*, 17(2): 165–79.

Fiske, S.T. (2018) Stereotype content: warmth and competence endure, *Current Directions in Psychological Science*, 27(2): 67–73.

Gewirtz-Meydan, A. and Ayalon, L. (2018) Forever young: visual representations of gender and age in online dating sites for older adults, *Journal of Women & Aging*, 30(6): 484–502.

Gewirtz-Meydan, A., Hafford-Letchfield, T., Benyamini, Y., Phelan, A., Jackson, J. and Ayalon, L. (2018) Ageism and sexuality, in L. Ayalon and C. Tesch-Roemer (eds) *Contemporary Perspectives on Ageism*, Springer, pp 149–62.

Hafford-Letchfield, T. (2008) What's love got to do with it? Developing supportive practices for the expression of sexuality, sexual identity and the intimacy needs of older people, *Journal of Care Services Management*, 2(4): 389–405.

Han, J. and Richardson, V.E. (2015) The relationships among perceived discrimination, self-perceptions of aging, and depressive symptoms: a longitudinal examination of age discrimination, *Aging & Mental Health*, 19(8): 747–55.

Hank, K. (2011) How 'successful' do older europeans age? Findings from SHARE, *Journals of Gerontology Series B: Psychological Sciences and Social Sciences*, 66(2): 230–6.

Hartley, H. (2006) The 'pinking'of Viagra culture: drug industry efforts to create and repackage sex drugs for women, *Sexualities*, 9(3): 363–78.

Heaphy, B. (2007) Sexualities, gender and ageing: resources and social change, *Current Sociology*, 55(2): 193–210.

Heredia, A.V. (2022) Feminism and pornography: from mainstream pornography (hetero-patriarchal) to post-porn (non-binary), *The Age of Human Rights Journal*, 18: 221–38.

Hinchliff, S. and Gott, M. (2008) Challenging social myths and stereotypes of women and aging: heterosexual women talk about sex, *Journal of Women & Aging*, 20(1–2): 65–81.

Hinchliff, S. and Gott, M. (2011) Seeking medical help for sexual concerns in mid-and later life: a review of the literature, *Journal of Sex Research*, 48(2–3): 106–17.

Hunter, M.M., Huang, A.J. and Wallhagen, M.I. (2020) 'I'm going to stay young': belief in anti-aging efficacy of menopausal hormone therapy drives prolonged use despite medical risks, *PloS One*, 15(5): e0233703.

Hurd, L., Mahal, R., Ng, S. and Kanagasingam, D. (2020) From invisible to extraordinary: representations of older LGBTQ persons in Canadian print and online news media, *Journal of Aging Studies*, 55: 100877.

Kenalemang, L.M. (2021) Visual ageism and the subtle sexualisation of older celebrities in L'Oréal's advert campaigns: a multimodal critical discourse analysis, *Ageing and Society*, 1–18.

Kenny, R. (2013) A review of the literature on sexual development of older adults in relation to the asexual stereotype of older adults, *Canadian Journal of Family and Youth/Le Journal Canadien de Famille et de la Jeunesse*, 5(1): 91–106.

Kotter-Grühn, D., Kleinspehn-Ammerlahn, A., Gerstorf, D. and Smith, J. (2009) Self-perceptions of aging predict mortality and change with approaching death: 16-year longitudinal results from the Berlin aging study, *Psychology and Aging*, 24(3): 654.

Krekula, C., Nikander, P. and Wilińska, M. (2018) Multiple marginalizations based on age: gendered ageism and beyond, in L. Ayalon and C. Tesch-Roemer (eds) *Contemporary Perspectives on Ageism*, Springer, Cham, pp 33–50.

Lamont, R.A., Swift, H.J. and Abrams, D. (2015) A review and meta-analysis of age-based stereotype threat: negative stereotypes, not facts, do the damage, *Psychology and Aging*, 30(1): 180.

Laumann, E.O., Glasser, D.B., Neves, R.C. and Moreira, E.D., Jr. (2009) A population-based survey of sexual activity, sexual problems and associated help-seeking behavior patterns in mature adults in the United States of America, *International Journal of Impotence Research*, 21(3): 171–8.

Lee, M.M., Carpenter, B. and Meyers, L.S. (2007) Representations of older adults in television advertisements, *Journal of Aging Studies*, 21(1): 23–30.

Lemish, D. and Muhlbauer, V. (2012) 'Can't have it all': representations of older women in popular culture', *Women & Therapy*, 35(3–4): 165–80.

Levy, B. (2009) 'Stereotype embodiment: a psychosocial approach to aging', *Current Directions in Psychological Science*, 18(6): 332–6.

Levy, B.R., Slade, M.D. and Kasl, S.V. (2002) 'Longitudinal benefit of positive self-perceptions of aging on functional health', *The Journals of Gerontology Series B: Psychological Sciences and Social Sciences*, 57(5): 409–17.

Levy, B.R., Chung, P.H., Bedford, T. and Navrazhina, K. (2014) Facebook as a site for negative age stereotypes, *The Gerontologist*, 54(2): 172–6.

Lindau, S.T. and Gavrilova, N. (2010) Sex, health, and years of sexually active life gained due to good health: evidence from two US population-based cross-sectional surveys of ageing, *British Medical Journal*, 340: c810.

Loos, E. and Ivan, L. (2018) Visual ageism in the media, in L. Ayalon and C. Tesch-Roemer (eds) *Contemporary Perspectives on Ageism*, Springer, Cham, pp 163–76.

Malta, S. (2007) Love actually! Older adults and their romantic internet relationships, *Australian Journal of Emerging Technologies and Society*, 5.

Mariano, J., Marques, S., Ramos, M.R., Gerardo, F., da Cunha, C.L., Girenko, A., Alexandersson, J., Stree, B., Lamanna, M., Lorenzatto, M., Mikkelsen, L.P., Bundgård-Jørgensen, U., Rêgo, S. and de Vries, H. (2021) Too old for technology? Stereotype threat and technology use by older adults, *Behaviour & Information Technology*, 1–12.

Marshall, B. (2008) Older men and sexual health: post-Viagra views of changes in function, *Generations*, 32(1): 21–7.

May, J. (2006) Secrets and lies: sex education and gendered memories of childhood's end in an Australian provincial city, 1930s–1950s, *Sex Education*, 6(1): 1–15.

McLaughlin, S.J., Connell, C.M., Heeringa, S.G., Li, L.W. and Roberts, J.S. (2010) Successful aging in the United States: prevalence estimates from a national sample of older adults, *Journals of Gerontology Series B: Psychological Sciences and Social Sciences*, 65(2): 216–26.

Meisner, B.A. (2021) Are you OK, Boomer? Intensification of ageism and intergenerational tensions on social media amid COVID-19, *Leisure Sciences*, 43(1–2): 56–61.

Minichiello, V., Rahman, S., Dune, T., Scott, J. and Dowsett, G. (2013) E-health: potential benefits and challenges in providing and accessing sexual health services, *BMC Public Health*, 13(1): 1–7.

Pew Research Center (2017) Technology use among seniors [online], Available from: https://www.pewresearch.org/internet/2017/05/17/technology-use-among-seniors/

Pew Research Center (2020) Americans' personal experiences with online dating [online], Available from: https://www.pewresearch.org/internet/2020/02/06/americans-personal-experiences-with-online-dating/

Price, J., Patterson, R., Regnerus, M. and Walley, J. (2016) How much more XXX is Generation X consuming? Evidence of changing attitudes and behaviors related to pornography since 1973, *Journal of Sexual Research*, 53(1): 12–20.

Rajendran, L. and Thesinghraja, P. (2014) The impact of new media on traditional media, *Middle-East Journal of Scientific Research*, 22(4): 609–16.

Roy, S. and Ayalon, L. (2020) Age and gender stereotypes reflected in Google's 'Autocomplete' function: the portrayal and possible spread of societal stereotypes, *The Gerontologist*, 60(6): 1020–8.

Sargent-Cox, K.A., Anstey, K.J. and Luszcz, M.A. (2012) The relationship between change in self-perceptions of aging and physical functioning in older adults, *Psychology and Aging*, 27(3): 750.

Sargent-Cox, K.A., Anstey, K.J. and Luszcz, M.A. (2014) Longitudinal change of self-perceptions of aging and mortality, *Journals of Gerontology Series B: Psychological Sciences and Social Sciences*, 69(2): 168–73.

Scandurra, C., Mezza, F., Esposito, C., Vitelli, R., Maldonato, N.M., Bochicchio, V., Chiodi, A., Giami, A., Valerio, P. and Amodeo, A.L. (2022) Online sexual activities in Italian older adults: the role of gender, sexual orientation, and permissiveness, *Sexuality Research and Social Policy*, 19(1): 248–63.

Sevcikova, A., Vašek, D., Blinka, L., Machackova, H. and Ježek, S. (2021) Markers of sexual life and health in association with internet use for sexual purposes in Czechs aged 50 and older, *Sexuality Research and Social Policy*, 18: 1–13.

Simpson, P., Wilson, C.B., Brown, L., Horne, M. and Dickinson, T. (2018) 'We've had our sex life way back': older care home residents, sexuality and intimacy, *Ageing & Society*, 38(7): 1478–501.

Simpson, P., Brown, L., Wilson, C.B., Dickinson, T., Horne, M. and Torkington, K. (2017) Old(er) care home residents and sexual/intimate citizenship, *Ageing & Society*, 37(2): 243–65.

Træen, B., Carvalheira, A., Kvalem, I. and Hald, G. (2018) European older adults' use of the internet and social networks for love and sex, *Cyberpsychology: Journal of Psychosocial Research on Cyberspace*, 12: 1.

Træen, B., Carvalheira, A., Kvalem, I.L., Štulhofer, A., Janssen, E., Graham, C.A., Hald, G.M. and Enzlin, P. (2017) Sexuality in older adults (65+): an overview of the recent literature, Part 2: body image and sexual satisfaction, *International Journal of Sexual Health*, 29(1): 11–21.

Wada, M., Clarke, L.H. and Rozanova, J. (2015) Constructions of sexuality in later life: Analyses of Canadian magazine and newspaper portrayals of online dating. *Journal of Aging Studies*, 32: 40–9.

Walz, T. (2002) Crones, dirty old men, sexy seniors: representations of the sexuality of older persons, *Journal of Aging and Identity*, 7(2): 99–112.

Wandke, H., Sengpiel, M. and Sönksen, M. (2012) Myths about older people's use of information and communication technology, *Gerontology*, 58(6): 564–70.

Watson, W. and Stelle, C. (2021) Love in cyberspace: self presentation and partner seeking in online dating advertisements of older adults, *Journal of Family Issues*, 42(10): 2438–63.

Whittaker, R. (1998) Re-framing the representation of women in advertisements for hormone replacement therapy, *Nursing Inquiry*, 5(2): 77–86.

Xu, W. (2021) *Ageism in the Media: Online Representations of Older People*, Unpublished Thesis, Linköping University Electronic Press.

8

Older internet dating: ageist prescriptions and novel resexualising

Christine Beasley and Mary Holmes

Introduction

Internet dating is a 'purposeful form of meeting new people through specifically designed internet sites', with online dating services increasingly targeting *all* age groups (Barraket and Henry-Waring, 2008: 149–50). In the wake of its growing usage, internet dating has become entangled in wider concerns regarding sexual and emotional marketisation and misuse of personal data by internet companies, as well as associated with deceit, fraud, harassment, abuse and rape (see for example Bogolyubova et al, 2018). Simultaneously it has been a site of hope, pleasure, joy and of course desire, romance and love, including for older people.

Dating sites for 'older people' (those over 50) are flourishing (Watson and Stelle, 2021), yet most literature on internet dating has ignored older daters in favour of the young (Huyck, 2020; see also McWilliams and Barrett, 2014: 412). The political nature of the term 'older' (King and Calasanti, 2013: 699) has led us to choose what seems the most inclusive, neutral and common categorisation among dating websites and apps: referring to all those over 50 years as 'older'. Older heterosexual daters are marginalised within the realm of heterosexual dating and thus offer potential insights into some of its fractures. Elsewhere we have argued that relations of dominance do not describe heterosexuality in its entirety (Beasley et al, 2012) and outlined how varying aspects of online dating demonstrate its heterodoxical possibilities (Beasley and Holmes, 2021). We deliberately attend to heterosexual accounts of internet dating because of our existing theoretical interests in exploring signs of social change within 'the realm of the dominant' (Beasley and Holmes, 2021: 84). In this context, we reject widely accepted views about heterosexuality as inevitably heteronormative. We explore innovative possibilities for social change, specifically in relation to troubling gendered heteronormativity and advancing gender equality.[1] In this chapter, foregrounding older heterosexual daters offers a lens on the variable nature of heterosexual relations and reveals potential for social change.

To examine older internet daters' experiences, we use Australian and UK online accounts of internet dating (Beasley and Holmes, 2021).[2] While we cannot know how representative they are of all daters in those countries,[3] the full sample contains a wide selection of stories about hundreds of dates told by at least 70 daters over the last 20 years. The accounts necessarily arise from those who are willing to share their experiences, but they do tell us what daters think it is important to communicate and many of those writing about their experiences are over 50. The accounts of dating include 'found' data written by daters themselves and data 'made' by researchers, journalists or other commentators featuring the voices of internet daters (Stanley and Sereva, 2019; for more details see Beasley and Holmes, 2021: 7–11). Although these are 'Western' examples of internet dating, we depart from the ubiquitous focus on North America (Kisilevich et al, 2012: 609).[4]

The increasing number of online dating services for older daters (Hogan et al, 2011) gives our investigation significance, especially given the lack of literature on the topic (Menkin et al, 2015; Field, 2018). Population ageing is accelerating and more people are living and being active for many years after retirement (Australian Productivity Commission, 2013: 33; Spijker and MacInnes, 2013; Office for National Statistics, 2019). However, most research on older online daters primarily concerns health risks (Brown and Shinohara, 2013), in keeping with wider tendencies to represent older people and their health, desirability and sexuality as deficient and in decline (Gewirtz-Meydan and Ayalon, 2018). The prevailing youth focus and associated relatively negative approach towards older internet daters provides a crucial imperative for an alternative direction signalling resexualising opportunities.

Since research on internet dating almost invariably privileges the young, it reproduces systemic prejudice against older people that discounts their complexity as human beings, as irreducibly social subjects, as relational and interconnected bodies, and as socio-political agents. More constructive perspectives are emerging but 'the view of old age as a defeated stage of life' (Kendig and McCallum, 1987: 59) persists. Moreover, internet dating often reiterates gendered heteronorms. Yet, this is not the whole story. We begin by challenging the deficit model of ageing. We then focus on reimagining possibilities concerning sexuality and intimacy, detailing quandaries associated with a critique of ageism and challenges to gendered heteronormativity. Finally, in reconsidering deficit models of ageing, we outline novel directions with regard to eroticism and intimate companionability that present older internet daters as practicing sexuality/intimacy in ways that are socially innovative. We ask overall whether heterosexual internet dating among older people offers opportunities for enhancing social equality.

Challenging the deficit model

Despite more constructive perspectives emerging, a deficit model of ageing remains prevalent, even where cultures respect elders (Sargent-Cox, 2017: 5; Vauclair et al, 2017; Qi, 2021: 54), and this model includes denying that older people are sexual beings. Ageist desexualisation also involves conceiving older adults as normatively distanced or disconnected from physical and emotional intimacy. Thus, to grasp the impact of ageism it is necessary to clarify terminologies around age, sexuality and intimacy. We conceive of sexuality as within the continuum of intimacy, but also as distinguishable from it (see also Reynolds et al, Series Editors' introduction). The term sexuality encompasses not merely sexual acts, practices and experiences but also a conglomerate of institutions, identities, social assumptions and customs, as well as resources and labour (Beasley and Holmes, 2021: 6). By comparison, intimacy usually refers to a more diffuse arena than sexuality, concerned with a sense of close, embodied and particularised personal connection (Jamieson, 1999; Beasley and Holmes, 2021: 6–7), as well as potentially involving affectionate touch (Debrot et al, 2013). Intimacy is typically not an individualised experience, but also embedded in relationalities (Smart, 2007). We consider sexuality and intimacy as linked, though not reducible to each other. Importantly, in the setting of this volume, we note that sexuality is not necessarily intimate, and that intimacy is not necessarily directly sexual in the sense of bodily intimacy and genital contact. More specifically, as our later examples show, we do not presume that intimacy without bodily closeness is therefore without sexualised elements, let alone that such connections are inevitably 'desexualised'.

The aim of the *Sex and Intimacy in Later Life* series, to which this volume belongs, is to counter deficit understandings of older people and to 'put the sex back into sexuality (and ageing)' (Series Editors' introduction). This requires a broad understanding of what counts as sexual. In keeping with the series editors' approach to Rennie's work in a previous volume of the series, we consider it is possible to 'retain the value of recognisable sexual pleasures while recognising that the balance of physical pleasure, emotional satisfaction and sensual practices may vary' (Series Editors' introduction). The trick is to avoid a delimited conception of sexuality and to maintain an expanded understanding of both sexuality and intimacy without erasing bodily contact and sex. This entails refusing neat divisions between 'resexualisation' and 'desexualisation' (Reynolds et al, 2021; Series Editors' introduction). Challenges to the desexualisation of older people may involve acknowledgement of sex and heterodoxical directions that reject 'ageist erotophobia', *as well as* other departures from ageist assumptions concerning intimacy and sexuality. Resexualising, in short, may not be particularly obviously physical/bodily. This point is significant in situating our analysis of older internet dating within a critique of ageism.

Ageism involves a deficit model of growing old that focuses on, and can contribute to, negative experiences in old age, such as diminishing health, independence and finances (Sargent-Cox, 2017). In the UK and Australia, older adults commonly lose status as they are thought to become isolated, frail burdens on families and societies (Officer et al, 2016: 710). Older people often internalise these stereotypes, which can negatively impact on their sexual interest and sexual activity (Heywood et al, 2019). Internet dating may not always challenge desexualised representations and expectations of ageing. Sometimes linking up online involves conventional ideas about romantic connections (Whitty, 2008), exhibiting 'sticky' affects and limiting efforts to escape social norms (Ahmed, 2007: 11, 60, 89–95; Beasley and Holmes, 2021: 15–33). Older women might, for instance, feel unable to contact men and sit waiting to receive messages (Frohlick and Migliardi, 2011: 79–81; McWilliams and Barrett, 2014: 422). Moreover, the policing of women's sexuality and bodies is ongoing and remains difficult to ignore even as women age.[5] Older women may, for example, continue to feel the need to work on their appearance to approach closer to youthful ideals of feminine sexual attractiveness. And it does seem that older men do expect some conformity to these ideals (McWilliams and Barrett, 2014: 416, 425; Gewirtz-Meydan and Ayalon, 2018). However, there are also signs of unassuming yet significant challenges to ageism arising in the experiences of older online daters.

Older users see online dating as a useful way to expand their opportunities for social contact, despite experiencing some problems (Vandeweerd et al, 2016). Lillian (62) says it provides a crucial, incommensurable means to be able to develop relationships with new people.

> You come home from work, you want to be talking to someone about your day, it's good for your mental health … For women of my generation you can't just walk into a pub by yourself. (Lillian, UK, online article, 2020)

Like Lillian, many users convey their pleasure in engaging with what they deem an accessible and effective technology of intimacy. As one older dater in Malta's (2007: 94) study puts it,

> I had virtually no luck offline. First, I have no idea how to meet men [because] I'd been married for a long time. Second, I'm not gorgeous, and hate being rejected out of hand. Using [this dating site] was amazingly easy.

These daters find talking with others online easy and gain affirmation of their social desirability, although what that means in sexual terms can vary. Thus, the degree to which internet dating enables heterodoxies requires more examination.

Ageism and bodily intimacy: heterodoxical quandaries

Some of the heterodoxies associated with older internet dating have the potential to challenge the ageist neglect of older adults' bodily/sexual intimacies. Both popular and scholarly literature represent older people as desexualised. This dehumanises older people and limits recognition of the heterodoxical possibilities contained in their practices, including internet dating practices. Research typically neglects older people's emotions, bodies and intimate relationships, or treats them with distaste. This neglect is evident in an ageist focus on the young in most studies on internet dating (Hillier et al, 2012; Beasley and Holmes, 2016: 205). What limited discussion exists about older people's internet dating says little about bodily intimacy, desire, sexuality and sexual practices and mostly covers a limited range of possible connections (although see Malta, 2007; Debrot et al, 2013; Malta and Farquharson, 2014; McWilliams and Barrett, 2014).

Existing literature on older internet daters is predominantly negative, like most sex research on older people. Studies tend to focus on problems such as loneliness, exposure to unwanted sexual content or to sexually transmitted diseases (despite the latter being a low risk) (Bateson et al, 2012; McWilliams and Barrett, 2014; Albury et al, 2020). What knowledge there is of ageing sexualities comes mainly from large-scale medically-oriented quantitative studies. We have little qualitative knowledge informed by older men and women voicing their understandings and experiences of sexuality (Sandberg, 2011: 264). This is partly because of normative expectations that older people are not sexual, and if they are sexually active this is deemed abnormal and even unseemly (Adams et al, 2003: 405; Malta, 2007: 84). Such ageism restricts our knowledge of everyday sexual understandings and practices among older people and reaffirms, rather than challenges, gendered heteronormativity (Fileborn et al, 2017: E41). Ageism thus leaves a gap in knowledge of what we call the 'micro-politics' of heterosexual internet dating (Beasley and Holmes, 2021: 3, 57; see also McWilliams and Barrett, 2014: 430), a gap that we have sought to fill through attention to older internet daters' modes of intimacy and sexuality.

Heterodoxical challenges to desexualisation

As noted earlier, our focus here is upon the implications of heterosexual online dating in relation to age and gender in terms of social change.

Although online daters over 50 may rarely enact more radical departures from sexual and relationship norms, their interactions with new technologies can enable some innovations around ageing, intimacy/sexuality, gender subjectivities and heteronormativity. These innovations might be more common among the young-old (50–74) (Alterovitz and Mendelsohn, 2013). Nevertheless, a good proportion of older people remain sexually active into their 80s and beyond, and many others would like to be active (Freak-Poli, 2020). Internet dating enables many older internet daters to meet sexual partners via the internet (Malta, 2007; Malta and Farquharson, 2014: 243). In this setting, older internet daters challenge ageist assumptions about losing interest in bodily intimacy/sexuality as one ages. In one Canadian study, over-50-year-old heterosexual women reported enjoying casual sexual encounters organised via internet dating sites (Frohlick and Migliardi, 2011: 79–83). Similarly, Australian dater Yvette (66) says sex is 'very important' and internet dating has 'opened [her] eyes to the fact that some men still find [her] quite "yummy"' (Australia, online magazine article, 2014). These instances offer alternatives to common representations of older adults as inevitably desexualised.

Internet dating can enable some older heterosexual women to subvert gender norms around sexuality by demonstrating enthusiasm for sex, including casual sex (Malta, 2007; Frohlick and Migliardi, 2011: 83). Some older men are 'surprised' (Martin, Australia, online magazine article, 2014) by women's assertiveness about wanting to have sex. Giles (68) said he 'certainly didn't expect women to come on so strong' (Australia, newspaper article, 2015). Alison (66) is one example of women meeting this surprise in a direct manner, explaining that after becoming a widow she was abstinent for a long time, but has now enthusiastically embraced internet dating's sexual opportunities.

> It is all a big adventure. As long as I am up front with myself and my partners, I reckon I can do what feels good and have a ball. No more fears of pregnancy, no more of those crazy messages like 'He'll think you're a slut' or 'He'll think you are too easy'. What a load of rubbish all that was. (Alison, Australia, newspaper article, 2015)

Some older women also use internet dating to upset typical gender hierarchies in which male partners are older (McKenzie, 2015), by connecting with younger men online (Alarie, 2019). Dedicated 'cougar' dating sites suggest a considerable market for pairing younger men with older women.[6] The 'cougar' label is usually applied to sexually empowered and assertive older women (30 to 60) who pursue younger men. The label therefore has limits in challenging normative desexualisation of older-old women, and the relationships are not without difficulties (Alarie, 2019). However, it envisions sexual agency for older women and may enable 50+ women to take up heterodoxical options in internet dating and elsewhere. Twice-divorced 53-year-old Kate noted that,

> [w]ith older blokes showing no interest in me, I figured my time was up. So imagine my surprise to find younger men seemed to like me … I treated the apps as a social experiment in the wide variety of people dating in the UK. (Kate, UK, newspaper article, 2018)

Kate's experiment departs further from sexual and gendered norms than younger women finding 'toyboys' because these displays of sexual agency by older women breach deeply held ageist conventions marking them as asexual.

Internet dating also appears to allow older men to expand their range of emotional and sexual communication (Rowntree, 2014). Older men often report their reasons for dating as associated with their emotional needs but, although they may benefit more than women from heterosexual coupledom (McIntosh et al, 2011: 70, 79), this does not always mean men expect women to attend to those needs. Sandberg (2013: 261–2) outlines how many older Swedish men (aged 67–87) say that as they have aged they have moved towards a more mutual and communicative conception of relationships that departs from 'hegemonic' forms of masculinity associated with gender inequality.[7] Examples in our study, include John (57) and Robin (66) who happily report finding new relationships online where they 'just talked and talked about everything', or they felt they could share their emotions without their partner 'judging' them (UK, online magazine article, 2016). The spread of such gentle modifications is notable because change is not only achieved by rebellions but also by small-scale refashionings that we have earlier described as 'micro-politics'.

Reimagining the (biomedical/bodily) deficit model

One aspect of micro-politics is revealed in the embodied experiences of older internet daters, indicating that gendered heteronormative assumptions about them are not simply reiterated (Malta et al, 2020). Older women may face new experiences associated with dating with some trepidation, but post-menopause is not the end of sexually novel possibilities and innovative responses. Megan notes that after a lumpy start, a variety of unexpected opportunities arose.

> How has my experience in dating changed since I started going through menopause? Well it's changed completely … The beginning of my menopause was the hardest bit. It was like I was possessed by another person … The second thing that changed was my libido … Also there

> was weight gain, so not feeling very sexy anymore, foggy brain, and this constant desire of living in my comfy pyjamas (sic).
>
> After starting to understand more about the menopause and my menopause symptom (sic) … I started to feel excited again about life again. I started to feel normal, like me again.
>
> And so I am now 53 … Regarding my sex life, it is different as well. It is harder to have an orgasm, and you don't get as 'wet' as before down there. What I realised is that you have to be true to your own body and know what makes you aroused … That's why after starting to use my lubricants everything changed.
>
> Generally speaking … [i]f I was in a relationship, it will be for all of the right reasons, good chemistry with someone on my wavelength … But if for now I am single that's fine too, I'm in a good relationship with me, I am enough. (Megan, UK, online blog, 2019)

Megan's account, along with those of other older women in our study, shows flexibility around dating, a sense that she is 'enough', which troubles traditional conceptions of hetero-femininity and the supreme status of hetero-sex and hetero-coupling. By contrast, scholarly literature and popular culture represent a medicalised emphasis on older women daters' low libidos and atrophied dry vaginas. Pharmaceutical and surgical rejuvenation are offered through hormone replacement, testosterone therapies and cosmetic surgery. These perspectives compare older women with their younger counterparts, thus reinforcing uncertainty about the former's attractiveness, and their desire and capacity for heterosexual sex – equated with penis-vagina intercourse (Sandberg, 2013: 264). By this means, men's penises and erections are often, dare we say, re-erected as central.

Older women (along with older men) do not necessarily display marked concerns about their bodies, despite possible trepidation about dating. One blog even suggests that 'women aged between 65 and 74 tend to be the most confident about their bodies when compared with other age groups' (Anonymous, UK, dating site advice blog, 2019). Moreover, Megan is not alone in finding that dating enabled her to develop forms of confidence associated with being an older woman.

> Post-menopausal women are actually quite a desirable lot: more confident than our younger sisters, clear about what we want and even attractive to younger men who like the fact that we're more comfortable in our own skin, even if that skin is a little crepey. Most of my dating friends have been out with younger men and in some cases substantially younger men.
>
> Dating has given me a chance to laugh, be carefree and connect with something I'd lost in myself … Maybe dating in your 50s isn't about

> love, companionship, orgasms or even passionate kisses. Maybe it's about feeling that your life is still opening up, not shutting down, and that you can choose which direction you want to take it in. (Caterina, UK, online blog, 2018)

Caterina discovered, after enjoying internet dating, that 'ageing is a privilege, not something to dread'.

Older women's embodied practices evidence a range of heterodoxical innovations. Menopause and beyond do not necessarily signify dispiriting decline, nor age-defying 'sexy senior' status. A more complex picture emerges of ageing as enabling new social directions perhaps less available to the young. To propose that older women might be the vanguard of societal transformations around gender and sexuality is a challenge to commonly accepted ideas of age, gender, heterosexuality and social change.

Older men's experiences of internet dating, like women's, reveal the limitations of a biomedical agenda. The reduction of older men's social and sexual health, intimacy and pleasure into sexual 'erectile functioning' effaces other ways of seeing masculinity and age, not related to penis-vagina intercourse (Sandberg, 2013: 264; Fileborn et al, 2017: 2098). Many older men's experiences are not dominated by sexual 'dysfunction', rather they challenge gendered heteronorms through increased regard for emotionality and communication with female partners, a considerably expanded range of understandings of pleasure and of sexual practices, and an accompanying sense of the advantages of ageing (DeLamater and Koepsel, 2015; Ménard et al, 2015). Sandberg (2013) describes this shift 'from the "fiery urges" of youth to the freedom of intimacy'. This is not a deficit model (Calasanti, 2004; Beasley, 2008, 2015; Lodge and Umberson, 2013). Instead, Sandberg's (2013: 271) older male participants experienced intimate relationships as 'taking new shapes' away from a goal oriented hetero-sex focused upon men's performance and orgasm and towards more open-ended and interactive expressions of intimacy. This enabled them to become 'better, more considerate lovers', enjoying better relationships with female partners. Martin (69) implies that this has been his experience: 'the middle-aged and mature woman is a very sexual individual who wants to go to bed and be stroked' (Australia, online magazine article, 2014). Such accounts do not appear to be entirely self-serving since mid-to-later life couples (Lodge and Umberson, 2012) report a decrease in frequency but an increase in the quality of sexual encounters (see also Ménard et al, 2015; Australian Seniors, 2019).

Loss of certainties around erections, and associated doubts regarding phallocentric social norms, might not always be a misfortune and a medical 'problem'. Ageing may produce 'erectile dissatisfaction' compared to youthful vigor, but does not entail inevitable dysfunction (Laumann and Waite, 2008). Such dissatisfaction arises from acceptance of ageist presumptions in which youth is the axiomatically superior standard. A conception of manliness as located in the penis and its 'performance' fuels dissatisfaction. However, as one of the sixtysomething participants makes clear in Australian research on conversations about sex in primary health care settings, 'sex' can encompass 'other things and [you can] pleasure each other in other ways [which] can actually create the intimacy that can be lost if you're not having … penile-vaginal [sex]' (Malta et al, 2020: 43). In this study older Australian men show a consistent and strong concern to stress mutual enjoyment and equality as making sex pleasurable (Malta et al, 2020; see also Hughes, 2011). Rather than a soft penis necessarily representing loss and decline, a renewed focus on touch, fondling, hugging, kissing, mutual or parallel masturbation, oral sex, sexual 'aids' and sex games suggests quietly subversive, even dissident, practices enabling an unshackling from the constraints of normative heterosexuality. Older men's experiences – whether they involve sexual desire and sexual activities or not – may provide creative heterodoxical models for connection and intimacy as well as for hetero-sex and hetero-coupledom.

Like older women, rather than older men being 'past it' they may have much to offer in rethinking sociality and social change; potential often facilitated by internet dating. Young men may be heavily policed to perform forms of hegemonic masculinity that replicate men's authority over women through reiterated practices associated with the centrality of the penis and its companion, the 'coital imperative' (Willis et al, 2018). By comparison, older men may well be freer to undertake new social/sexual directions. As older dater Brian points out, 'the majority of senior single members have faced major change!' (Australia, online dating site advice blog, no date). Indeed, men over 50, along with their female counterparts, may defy expectations and unexpectedly be at the forefront of social change around gender and sexuality.

Contesting intimacy and sexuality: resexualisation and other directions

In critiquing the desexualisation of older people, we thus refuse 'ageist erotophobia' (Simpson et al, 2017), while opening up expanded notions of what counts as sexual and challenging conventional understandings of older people's experiences of intimacy. Nonconformity among older daters broadens understandings of the 'resexualising' of later life. One example is divergence from online dating's central focus on the goal of romantic/sexual hetero-coupledom into either personal development or various versions of platonic relationships. These options are not necessarily 'desexualised' and hence can be part of calls to acknowledge or enable resexualisation. They allow an expanded conception of challenges to ageism undertaken by older people that, even in the absence of overt eroticism or bodily sexual acts, exist on a spectrum of 'sexual' experiences.

There can be sexualised elements in using internet dating as a means to personal development (McWilliams and Barrett, 2014; Erjavec and Fiser, 2016: 366; Vandeweerd et al, 2016). Patsy, (65) says that after online dating for 8 years,

> I haven't minded [not meeting anyone] … I'm adding interest and variety to my life by having contact with people I wouldn't meet any other way. Anything else is a bonus. (Patsy, Australia, newspaper article, 2018)

For Patsy and many other older daters, making her life more interesting by meeting others does not amount to resexualisation in the strict sense, but expanded versions of sexuality can enfold this seeking of excitement, connection and intimacy with others.

Additionally, our study found heterodox possibilities arising from various kinds of platonic but powerful intimacies formed between older internet daters (Beasley and Holmes, 2021: see chapters 5 and 6). Here we focus on the formation of platonic relationships (which may have sexualised/eroticised elements but nevertheless offer intense platonic companionship) and cross-sex friendships. These options may in practice be difficult to distinguish, but both involve unconventional departures from hetero-sex and hetero-coupledom, undoing and redefining usual understandings of sexuality and intimacy and disrupting ageist assumptions about desexualisation. The emergence of such unorthodox 'partnering' is largely unheralded in discussions of internet dating. Platonic companionship is a more radically dissident partnership not centrally organised around fun, friendship or sexual connection. It is more emotionally intense, significant, committed and intimate than is considered 'normal' for a relationship built on casual enjoyment or friendship and provides ongoing companionable coupledom. Yet, it does not resemble the heteronormative standard for a romantic-sexual couple (Smith, 2018). We describe this non-normative coupledom as 'alternative-platonic' (AP) – rather than employing the language of 'queer' which most often denotes an 'opposition to hegemonic norms', a protest against the 'normal' (Showden, 2012: 8). The development of cross-sex AP relationships can be particularly important to older daters.

> One of my friends met several older gentlemen through online dating sites after her husband died. She had platonic relationships with a couple of them, eventually become cruise companions! (sic) … she enjoyed the company. (Beatrice, UK, advice article on social networking site, no date)

Beatrice notes the importance of platonic relationships for her friend. Cross-sex friendships are a similarly unconventional option, one that usually faces social disapproval. Such friendships are deemed impossible in the absence of equality and the 'obvious' differences between genders, thought to mask sexual repression, or to threaten heterosexual partnerships (Kalmijn, 2002). These friendships are typically taboo because they threaten gender distinction and identities and the ways in which these underpin heteronormative, and cultural, prescriptions about 'proper' relationships (Chaudhry, 2022). When over 50-year-olds use internet dating to make cross-sex friendships, they are subverting gendered heteronorms. Older women in particular may choose such friendships over more traditional heterosexual relationships, preferring companionship to loss of independence (McIntosh et al, 2011: 77–9; McWilliams and Barrett, 2014: 415, 420, 423–4; Vandeweerd et al, 2016). Older men might be keener than their women peers to have the safety and support of romantic hetero-coupledom (McWilliams and Barrett, 2014: 424–5), but they also enter different kinds of relationships via internet dating. For example, although Nigel (71) has not resigned from pursuing 'romantic relationships', he has enjoyed making cross-sex friendships.

> Obviously one has to be persistent and incredibly optimistic, but from my point of view I have had seven happy years, made some wonderful and permanent friends and lost nothing along the way. (Nigel, Australia, online magazine article, 2014)

Nigel is happy to have made friends, and many older daters are looking for a range of companions (Australian Seniors, 2019), rather than necessarily pursuing love and long-term relationships as dating sites expect. Indeed, few of the relationships made by over 60s online lead to cohabitation or marriage (Malta and Farquharson, 2014; Erjavec and Fiser, 2016: 362). Although most dating sites/apps 'are geared towards romance', this is not how most older adults apparently use them. Both the online dating industry and academic research tend to ignore these desires for cross-sex friendships, which provide one of a number of unexpected examples of older people taking the lead on socially transformative practices.

Concluding alternative perspectives

Prevalent ageism almost invariably links being older with a range of unappetising characteristics (Heywood et al, 2019) and deems older people without interest because they are seen as 'looking backwards rather than forwards' (Laurel, UK, online newspaper story, 2016). They are linked to closed-mindedness and social quietism. However, as this chapter shows, older adults' engagement in online dating illustrates a variety of examples of social innovation. There is much to indicate that far from being immured in social quietism, they are contributors to change.

Internet dating demonstrates much that remains normative. Nonetheless, our focus upon older people and intimacy/sexuality reveals many heterodox innovations that are politically significant when considering social change with regard to gendered heteronormativity. Daters over 50 are not inevitably frail, senile, and unattractive, let alone boring, but rather an un-recognised resource for re-imagining social, intimate and sexual life.

Notes

1. 'Heteronormativity' is a term that draws together a conception of heterosexuality as the natural, normal and best form of sexuality with a notion of an abiding gender binary in which there are only two forms of selfhood that are different and necessarily complementary (see Warner, 1999). Thus heterosexuality, heterosexual power relations, gender polarity and gendered power relations seem given, unquestionable and innate (Beasley et al, 2012: 3–5, 12, 22–3; Beasley and Holmes, 2019: 14). However, we are conscious that when the term is used, the axis of gender is sometimes less evident and hence throughout the chapter we have referred to 'gendered heteronormativity' to render its interwoven meaning in relation to gender, as well as sexuality, more visible.
2. For example, internet daters in China are apparently much more likely to be seeking marriage than those in the UK and Australia (Li and Lipscomb, 2017) and internet dating has been slower to gain acceptance and popularity in a range of countries including China (Xiao and Qian, 2020; Beasley and Holmes, 2021: 139–72).
3. Detailed information about methods and sources are available in our book (Beasley and Holmes, 2021); here we refer to the online accounts we analysed by giving the name of the person, their location, the type of source and year of posting online. For example, (Lillian, UK, online article, 2020).
4. In previous work our primary focus on UK and Australian internet daters is augmented by analysis of online dating in Denmark, Uganda, Argentina, China and Turkey.
5. There is a vast literature devoted to the historically deeply established control of women's bodies and sexuality in Western and indeed most cultures (Smart and Smart, 1978; Khanna and Price, 1994; Fischer and Seidman, 2016).
6. There are a range of definitions of the term 'cougar', but most refer to middle-aged women who date or wish to date significantly younger men – for example, younger men who are 10 years their junior (see Lawton and Callister, 2010: 6–7).
7. Within the field of critical studies in men and masculinities, Raewyn Connell's terminology of 'hegemonic masculinity' is virtually omnipresent and is a means to recognising that not all masculinities are equal. Rather, hegemonic masculinity offers an honoured and mobilising model of manliness to which all men are supposed to aspire and which is crucially defined by its function in legitimating gendered power relations, specifically men's power over women (Beasley, 2008: 88–9; see also Beasley et al, 2012).

References

Adams M., Oye, J. and Parker, T. (2003) Sexuality of older adults and the internet: from sex education to cybersex, *Sexual and Relationship Therapy*, 18(3): 405–15.

Ahmed, S. (2007) *The Cultural Politics of Emotion*, Routledge.

Alarie, M. (2019) 'They're the ones chasing the cougar': relationship formation in the context of age-hypogamous intimate relationships, *Gender & Society*, 33(3): 463–85.

Albury, K. McCosker, A., Pym, T. and Byron, P. (2020) Dating apps as public health 'problems': cautionary tales and vernacular pedagogies in news media, *Health Sociology Review*, 29(3): 232–48.

Alterovitz, S. and Mendelsohn, G. (2013) Relationship goals of middle-aged, young-old, and old-old internet daters: an analysis of online personal ads, *Journal of Aging Studies*, 27(2): 159–65.

Australian Productivity Commission (2013) An Ageing Australia: Preparing for the Future, Productivity Commission Research Paper, November [online], Available from: https://www.pc.gov.au/research/completed/ageing-australia/ageing-australia.pdf

Australian Seniors (2019) *Modern Dating* [online], Available from: https://www.seniors.com.au/news-insights/australian-seniors-series-modern-dating.

Barraket, J. and Henry-Waring, M. (2008) Getting it on (line): sociological perspectives on e-dating, *Journal of Sociology*, 44(2): 149–65.

Bateson, D.J., Weisberg, E., McCaffery, K.J. and Luscombe, G. (2012) When online becomes offline: attitudes to safer sex practices in older and younger women using an Australian internet dating service, *Sexual Health*, 9(2): 152–9.

Beasley, C. (2008) The challenge of pleasure: re-imagining sexuality and sexual health, *Health Sociology Review*, 17(2): 151–63.

Beasley, C. (2015) Libidinal heterodoxy: heterosexuality, hetero-masculinity and 'transgression'. *Men and Masculinities*, 18(2): 140–58.

Beasley, C. and Holmes, M. (2016) Internet dating, sexual intimacy and older people, in R. Harding and E. Peel (eds) *Ageing and Sexualities: Interdisciplinary Perspectives*, Ashgate, pp 205–22.

Beasley, C. and Holmes, M. (2021) *Internet Dating: Intimacy and Social Change*, Routledge.

Beasley, C., Brook, H. and Holmes, M. (2012) *Heterosexuality in Theory and Practice*, Routledge.

Bogolyubova, P., Panicheva, R., Tikhonov, V., Ivanov, V. and Ledovaya, Y. (2018) Dark personalities on Facebook: harmful online behaviors and language, *Computers in Human Behavior*, 78: 151–9.

Brown, S. and Shinohara, S. (2013) Dating relationships in older adulthood: a national portrait, *Journal of Marriage and Family*, 75(5): 1194–202.

Calasanti, T. (2004) Feminist gerontology and old men, *The Journals of Gerontology Series B: Psychological Sciences and Social Sciences*, 59(6): S305–14.

Chaudhry, S. (2022) Mid-and later life cross-sex friendships in minority ethnic contexts: insights from Scotland, *Sociological Research Online*, 27(4): 947–63.

Debrot, A., Schoebi, D., Perrez, M. and Horn, A. (2013) Touch as an interpersonal emotion regulation process in couples' daily lives: the mediating role of psychological intimacy, *Personality and Social Psychology Bulletin*, 39(10): 1373–85.

DeLamater, J. and Koepsel, E. (2015) Relationships and sexual expression in later life: a biopsychosocial perspective, *Sexual and Relationship Therapy*, 30(1): 37–59.

Erjavec, K. and Fiser, S. (2016) Aging adults about online dating: 'I am back on the relationship market!', *Polish Sociological Review*, 195: 361.

Field, T. (2018) Online dating profiles and problems in older adults: A review, *OBM Geriatrics*, 2(3), DOI: 10.21926/obm.geriatr.1803012

Fileborn, B., Lyons, A., Hinchliff, S., Brown, G., Heywood, W., Dow, B., Malta, S. and Minichiello, V. (2017) Improving the sexual lives of older Australians: perspectives from a qualitative study, *Australasian Journal on Ageing*, 36(4): E36–42.

Fischer, N.L. and Seidman, S. (2016) *Introducing the New Sexuality Studies* (3rd edition), Routledge.

Freak-Poli, R. (2020) It's not age that prevents sexual activity later in life, *Australasian Journal on Ageing*, 39(S1): 22–9.

Frohlick, S. and Migliardi, P. (2011) Heterosexual profiling online: online dating and 'becoming' heterosexualities for women aged thirty and older in the digital era, *Australian Feminist Studies*, 26(67): 73–88.

Gewirtz-Meydan, A. and Ayalon, L. (2018) Forever young: visual representations of gender and age in online dating sites for older adults, *Journal of Women & Aging*, 30(6): 484–502.

Heywood, W., Minichiello, V., Lyons, A., Fileborn, B., Hussain, R., Hinchliff, S., Malta, S., Barrett, C. and Dow, B. (2019) The impact of experiences of ageism on sexual activity and interest in later life, *Ageing & Society*, 39(4): 795–814.

Hillier, L., Mitchell, K. and Ybarra, M. (2012) The internet as a safety net: findings from a series of online focus groups with LGB and non-LGB young people in the United States, *Journal of LGBT Youth*, 9(3): 225–46.

Hogan, B., Li, N. and Dutton, W. (2011) *A Global Shift in the Social Relationships of Networked Individuals: Meeting and Dating Online Comes of Age*, Oxford Internet Institute.

Hughes, J. (2011) Are older men taking sexuality as prescribed? The implications of the competing influences on ageing male heterosexuality, *Australian Feminist Studies*, 26: 89–102.

Huyck, M. (2020) Falling in love in later life, in A. Abela, S. Vella and S. Piscopo (eds) *Couple Relationships in a Global Context: Understanding Love and Intimacy Across Cultures*, Springer, pp 177–91.

Jamieson, L. (1999) Intimacy transformed? A critical look at the 'pure relationship', *Sociology*, 33(3): 477–94.

Kalmijn, M. (2002) Sex segregation of friendship networks. Individual and structural determinants of having cross-sex friends, *European Sociological Review*, 18(1): 101–17.

Kendig, H. and McCallum, J. (1987) *Greying Australia: Future Impacts of Population Ageing*, Australian Government Publishing Service.

Khanna, R. and Price, J. (1994) Female sexuality, regulation and resistance, *Focus on Gender* (Population and Reproductive Rights), 2(2): 29–34.

King, N. and Calasanti, T (2013) Men's aging amidst intersecting relations of inequality, *Sociology Compass*, 7(9): 699–710.

Kisilevich, S., Ang, C. and Last, M. (2012) Large-scale analysis of self-disclosure patterns among online social networks users: a Russian context, *Knowledge and Information Systems*, 32(3): 609–28.

Laumann, E. and Waite, L. (2008) Sexual dysfunction among older adults: prevalence and risk factors from a nationally representative US probability sample of men and women 57–85 years of age, *The Journal of Sexual Medicine*, 5(10): 2300–11.

Lawton, Z. and Callister, P. (2010) Older women – younger men relationships: The social phenomenon of 'cougars'. A research note. Victoria University of Wellington, New Zealand: Institute of Policy Studies Working Paper 10/02, January.

Li, J. and Lipscomb, A. (2017) Love on the cloud: the rise of online dating in China, US-China Institute, *US-China Today*, 17 July.

Lodge, A. and Umberson, D. (2012) All shook up: sexuality of mid- to later life married couples, *Journal of Marriage and Family*, 74(3): 428–43.

Lodge, A. and Umberson, D. (2013) Age and embodied masculinities: midlife gay and heterosexual men talk about their bodies, *Journal of Aging Studies*, 27(3): 225–32.

Malta, S. (2007) Love actually! Older adults and their romantic internet relationships, *Australian Journal of Emerging Technologies and Society*, 5(2): 84–102.

Malta, S. and Farquharson, K. (2014) The initiation and progression of late-life romantic relationships, *Journal of Sociology*, 50(3): 237–51.

Malta, S., Temple-Smith, M., Bickerstaffe, A., Bourchier, L. and Hocking, J. (2020) 'That might be a bit sexy for somebody your age': older adult sexual health conversations in primary care, *Australasian Journal on Ageing*, 39: 40–8.

McIntosh, W.D., Locker, L., Briley, K., Ryan, R. and Scott, A. (2011) What do older adults seek in their potential romantic partners? Evidence from online personal ads, *The International Journal of Aging and Human Development*, 72(1): 67–82.

McKenzie, L. (2015) *Age-Dissimilar Couples and Romantic Relationships: Ageless Love?* Palgrave Macmillan.

McWilliams, S. and Barrett, A. (2014) Online dating in middle and later life: gendered expectations and experiences, *Journal of Family Issues*, 35(3): 411–36.

Ménard, A., Kleinplatz, P., Rosen, L., Lawless, S., Paradis, N., Campbell, M. and Huber, J.D. (2015) Individual and relational contributors to optimal sexual experiences in older men and women, *Sexual and Relationship Therapy*, 30(1): 78–93.

Menkin, J., Robles, T., Wiley, J. and Gonzaga, G. (2015) Online dating across the life span: users' relationship goals, *Psychology and Aging*, 30(4): 987–93.

Office for National Statistics (2019) *National Life Tables, UK: 2016–2018* [online], Available from: https://www.ons.gov.uk/peoplepopulationandcommunity/birthsdeathsandmarriages/lifeexpectancies/bulletins/nationallifetablesunitedkingdom/2016to2018.

Officer, A., Schneiders, M., Wu, D., Nash, P. Thiyagarajan, J.A. and Beard, J.R. (2016) Valuing older people: time for a global campaign to combat ageism, *Bulletin of the World Health Organisation*, 94: 710–10A.

Qi, X. (2021) *Remaking Families in Contemporary China*, Oxford University Press.

Reynolds, P., Simpson, P. and Hafford-Letchfield, T. (2021) *Sex and Diversity in Later Life: Critical Perspectives*, Policy Press.

Rowntree, M. (2014) 'Comfortable in my own skin': a new form of sexual freedom for ageing baby boomers, *Journal of Aging Studies*, 31: 150–8.

Sandberg, L. (2011) *Getting Intimate: A Feminist Analysis of Old Age, Masculinity and Sexuality*, Unpublished PhD Thesis. Linköping University, Sweden.

Sandberg, L. (2013) Just feeling a naked body close to you: men, sexuality and intimacy in later life, *Sexualities*, 16(3/4): 261–82.

Sargent-Cox, K. (2017) Ageism: we are our own worst enemy? *International Psychogeriatrics*, 29(1): 1–8.

Showden, C. (2012) Theorising maybe: A feminist/queer theory convergence, *Feminist Theory*, 13(1): 3–25.

Simpson, P., Brown, L.J.E., Wilson, C.B., Dickinson, T., Horne, M. and Torkington, K. (2017) Old(er) care home residents and sexual/intimate citizenship, *Ageing & Society*, 37(2), 243–65.

Smart, C. (2007) *Personal Life: New Directions in Sociological Thinking*, Polity.

Smart, C. and Smart, B. (eds) (1978) *Women, Sexuality and Social Control*, Routledge and Kegan Paul.

Smith, L. (2018) What is a quasiplatonic aka queerplatonic relationship? 18 April [online], Available from: https://www.pinknews.co.uk/2018/04/18/what-is-a-quasiplatonic-aka-queerplatonic-friendship/.

Spijker, J. and MacInnes, J. (2013) Population ageing: the timebomb that isn't? *The British Medical Journal*, 347: f6598.

Stanley, L. and Sereva, E. (2019) Documents of life: in theory and practice, in P. Atkinson, S. Delamont, A. Cernat, J. Sakshaug and R. Williams (eds) *SAGE Research Methods. Foundations*, Sage.

Vandeweerd, C., Myers, J., Coulter, M., Yalcin, A. and Corvin, J. (2016) Positives and negatives of online dating according to women 50+, *Journal of Women & Aging*, 28(3): 259–70.

Vauclair, C.-M., Hanke, K., Huang, L.-L. and Abrams, D. (2017) Are Asian cultures really less ageist than Western ones? It depends on the questions asked, *International Journal of Psychology*, 52(2): 136–44.

Warner, M. (1999) *The Trouble with Normal: Sex, Politics and the Ethics of a Queer Life*, Harvard University Press.

Watson, W. and Stelle, C. (2021) Love in cyberspace: self presentation and partner seeking in online dating advertisements of older adults, *Journal of Family Issues*, 42(10): 2438–63.

Whitty, M.T. (2008) Liberating or debilitating? An examination of romantic relationships, sexual relationships and friendships on the net, *Computers in Human Behavior*, 24(5): 1837–50.

Willis, M., Jozkowski, K.N., Lo, W. and Sanders, S.A. (2018) Are women's orgasms hindered by phallocentric imperatives?, *Archives of Sexual Behaviour*, 47: 1565–76.

Xiao, S. and Qian, Y. (2020) Mate selection among online daters in Shanghai: why does education matter? *Chinese Journal of Sociology*, 6(4): 521–46.

9

Resexualisation of older adults through sex care services in Dutch nursing homes

Nathalie Huitema and Tineke Roelofs

Introduction

Ambiguous attitudes toward sexuality and ageing are strongly embedded in Western society, as they are in the Netherlands, and are reinforced through myths and stereotypes. This neglect of the sexuality of older adults is even more true for older adults with potentially multiple disabilities and cognitive impairments – for example, those caused by dementia. When these impairments increase, living at home becomes impossible, and admission into a nursing home becomes inevitable. People then receive the highly intensive, specialised care they need within these nursing homes. However, this also implies a significant dependency on formal caregivers and staff in all parts of life, including the need to fulfil intimate and sexual needs. The myths and the stereotypes around sexuality and older adults have desexualised this group, as there's a societal view that older adults are asexual or lack sexual desire altogether.

Researchers have attempted to normalise sexuality and emphasise the importance of sexuality for nursing home residents (Mahieu and Gastmans, 2015; Roelofs et al, 2015; Syme, 2014), primarily by reporting on the perspectives of care staff and management along with the observed behaviour of residents.[1] In recent years, the resident perspective has increasingly become the point of interest (Bauer et al, 2013; Roelofs et al, 2021). This research revealed that the need for intimacy and sexuality was always present in nursing home residents. However, as older adults are commonly considered asexual, their sexual expression is often interpreted as inappropriate behaviour. This is not a complete misconception, as sexual behaviour in residents with dementia can result from different aspects. A natural, and normal need for sexuality is one, but also disinhibition resulting from severe cognitive disability occurs. Consequently, older nursing home residents face numerous barriers to experiencing sexuality (Roelofs et al, 2021), including practical and privacy barriers.

Dutch nursing homes in general have been becoming increasingly aware of the importance of sexuality in the lives of older adults. Due to the implementation of person-centred care (PCC) as the leading care paradigm, care is more and more focused on increasing quality of life, which in turn makes it impossible to ignore the need for sexuality. This awareness means that an increasing number of nursing homes have developed sexuality guidelines, and offer specialised training for staff. Some nursing homes even include sex workers in the options that are available for their residents. We consider this movement towards normalising all aspects of a residents' sexual needs as part of resexualisation of older adults who are dependent on nursing home care.

The inclusion of sex services in Dutch nursing homes is slowly gaining ground, and an increasing number of nursing home organisations acknowledge the need for intimacy and sexuality provisions for their residents. In the Netherlands, at least 15 per cent of nursing home residents admit that they miss intimacy in some way (Kuyper et al, 2018), and many residents state they miss 'being together' (Roelofs et al, 2021, 2019). As nursing home organisations started to aim for the fulfillment of the needs of their residents, professional sex worker organisations have developed, focusing exclusively on providing sex work to residents with disabilities and cognitive impairments. Historically and culturally, the Netherlands has been at the forefront of innovation and open-mindedness about sexuality, as seen through the example of legalised general sex work. However, the inclusion of sexual services in nursing home care is still a rarity.

In the Netherlands, there exists a specialised group of sex workers who cater exclusively to young and older adults dependent on care. These professionals, whom we refer to as 'sex care workers', possess additional knowledge of disabilities and cognitive impairments, with many having a background in nursing or social work within long term care (LTC) facilities. Sex care workers have specialised experience and knowledge regarding individuals with disabilities or cognitive impairments and typically spend more time with their clients per session. They focus on building a relationship with their clients, creating a comfortable and trusting environment. They maintain their expertise through additional courses and intervision groups. Beyond their primary role, they attend to extra needs, such as creating a comfortable environment for the client, and taking the time to ease the client's comfort.

This chapter does not discuss the morality of and justification for sex care work in general, nor does it discuss sex trafficking. Moreover, we do not implicitly or explicitly discuss gender orientation or sexual orientation, as we consider intimate and sexual needs as present in all people. Rather, we highlight how former healthcare workers became specialists in providing intimate and sexual support to ageing residents and centre the positive effects of this service on nursing home residents and the people who take care of them.

The nursing home care system in the Netherlands

Healthcare in the Netherlands is provided through a universal public health insurance program operated by semi-private health insurers and healthcare providers. All residents are entitled to a comprehensive basic health insurance package. Notably, nearly all health insurance companies in the Netherlands are not-for-profit cooperatives, allocating profits to required reserves or returning them as lower premiums. Moreover, nursing home care is laid down in law for every individual resident (Wet Langdurige Zorg (WLZ), 2024).

Consequently, socioeconomic status does not affect the quality of healthcare received, even though some people pay more through an income-dependent personal contribution. The Dutch long-term healthcare system is primarily government-funded, ensuring accessibility for everyone needing LTC. The number of private LTC facilities is limited, resulting in a wide range of socioeconomic statuses among residents in public LTC facilities. Financially, almost every aspect of care is covered in nursing home care. However, sex care services are not currently included.

Nursing home care is exclusively set up for people with severe disabilities and impairments who can no longer reside at home, even with formal care. Dutch nursing home care is more and more based on a PCC approach, focusing on general well-being, potential and quality of life (QoL). Nursing home care is divided into three main categories based on residents' care needs. In the first category, people with severe somatic disabilities live in open somatic care units. Although these residents receive 24-hour intensive physical care, they are able and allowed to leave the nursing home to run errands or visit family and friends. The second category consists of special psychogeriatric units for residents with moderate to severe dementia. These units are generally semi-closed units where residents cannot leave the facility on their own, and they are guided and cared for around the clock. Finally, the third category are geriatric rehabilitation units, where people who need rehabilitation after surgery, illness or stroke reside and receive specialised treatment temporarily.

Nursing homes' resexualisation requirements

Resexualisation in nursing home settings involves rethinking and redesigning the care environment to address the personal preferences and needs of highly dependent residents. Critical requirements for successful implementation include adopting PCC, providing comprehensive sexuality training for staff, establishing explicit sexuality guidelines and policies, and, if possible, employing a part-time sexologist.

These requirements not only focus on individual residents but also optimise the social environment, aligning with the selective optimization and compensation (SOC) theory (Baltes and Baltes, 1990). This theory considers resident-centred needs, strengths and limits to selectively compensate and optimise conditions, ensuring a holistic enhancement of residents' quality of life. Failure to meet these requirements will likely impede the resexualisation of older adults in nursing homes. The following sections will detail these requirements and their significance.

National legalisation

Sex work has been legal in the Netherlands for centuries. Currently, sex workers are legally identified as independent workers with all the rights and obligations that come with that, such as paying income tax and receiving a state pension at the age of 65.

Person-centred care

The developing body of research concerning intimacy and sexuality in LTC goes alongside another paradigm change in the context of nursing homes: moving away from the medical model, where preservation of health, safety and longevity were the main goal of care, towards a PCC model of care (Koren, 2010). This care paradigm provides a conceptual rationale in which intimacy and sexuality are logically, however often not explicitly, included. Although international literature provides different definitions of PCC, there is a consensus on PCC as a holistic, biopsychosocial model of care that aims to retain or improve the quality of life, dignity and well-being of residents (McCormack, 2004; Koren, 2010; Fazio et al, 2018). This paradigm focuses on gaining an understanding of the experiences, needs and values of residents to give them a voice and enable shared decision-making. In practice, this includes offering choices to residents concerning personal matters, such as determining their own food choices, care preferences and bedtimes (Koren, 2010). According to Fazio et al (2018), PCC has psychosocial benefits for residents and staff, such as decreased agitation and improved QoL for residents and reduced stress among staff members. As a consequence of this paradigm change, very personal aspects of life such as love, intimacy and sexuality could no longer be ignored in the nursing home, and an increasing emphasis was brought to the benefits of intimate and sexual expression (Roelofs et al, 2021). Moreover, in the Netherlands, quality of care ratings are increasingly based on the resident perspective (Sion et al, 2020). This results in nursing home organisations including residents' perspectives more often in policy and care planning related to residents' needs for intimacy and sexuality.

Sexuality training

Nursing home staff training in sexuality is crucial in nursing home care, as it significantly improves staff attitudes and reduces stigma (Di Napoli et al, 2013). Encouragingly, studies by Chen et al (2017) and Mahieu et al (2016) show that staff are generally supportive of receiving education about late-life sexuality. This is particularly important given the pervasive lack of knowledge about sexuality issues and dementia among nursing staff, often leading to sexual illiteracy. Increased training enhances staff knowledge and fosters more positive attitudes, creating a more supportive environment for residents' sexual expression. Training increases the understanding of the complexities of internal decision-making processes, influenced by factors such as residents' families (Waterschoot et al, 2022). Without proper training, staff may struggle to categorise sexual behavior appropriately, often influenced by personal and cultural values. Thus, implementing comprehensive training and sexual literacy policies can help staff differentiate between residents' rights and their need for sexual intimacy, ultimately reducing the impact of individualised values on sexual behavior.

Sexuality guidelines/policy

Having sexuality-focused policies in nursing home care is essential for improving staff attitudes towards residents' sexual desires and needs. Thys et al (2019) highlight that clear guidelines significantly influence staff behaviour and attitudes, while the lack of such policies underscores the urgent need for a human-rights-based approach to dementia care. Policies addressing intimacy and sexuality in LTC benefit staff, residents, and their families by providing necessary guidance. Doll (2013) notes that the absence of policies often leads staff to view sexual behaviour as problematic. Research by Tzeng et al (2009) and Thys et al (2019) shows that institutional policies directly affect staff attitudes, with liberal guidelines fostering open-mindedness. Staff themselves acknowledge the need for more direction in managing residents' sexual expression (Di Napoli et al, 2013), as without formal policies, nurses tend to adopt a conservative approach, which can be less accommodating to residents' sexual needs and rights (Vandrevala et al, 2017).

Sexologist

The first author of this chapter was the pioneering sexologist working in nursing home care in the Netherlands. Over the years, more sexologists focused on older adults, and nursing home care sexology emerged; in addition, some psychologists working in LTC completed their dissertations on sexuality in LTC. These pioneers not only significantly changed the nursing home landscape, but also supported the resexualisation of LTC by focusing on intimacy and sexuality as essential aspects of overall well-being and quality of life.

The evolution of sex care work in the Netherlands

Historically, only regular sex workers provided sexual services in LTC. However, these workers often lacked familiarity with the physical disabilities and cognitive impairments prevalent among LTC residents, leading to concerns about exploitation and unreliability for an already vulnerable group (Koenders, 2021). After incidents where residents didn't get what they paid for or even got robbed, the residents of a specialised village for individuals with physical disabilities developed a new model for sexual services. This model led to the establishment of Stichting Alternatieve Relatiebemiddeling [Alternative Relationship Mediation Foundation] (SAR) in 1982, a non-profit organisation specialising in sexual care services for people with disabilities (SAR, n.d.). Initially, the sex services were provided exclusively by and for people with physical disabilities, but the scope later expanded to include young individuals with mental and cognitive disabilities and older adults with physical and cognitive impairments in LTC.

Later, similar focused sex care organisations were founded and currently, approximately 100 specialised sex care workers operate in the Netherlands, catering to the disabled and ageing populations. Sex care workers encompass a range of activities beyond intercourse, including instruction on masturbation and providing emotional support (Nwanazia, 2018). These sex care organisations maintain strict staff-selection processes to ensure professionalism and competence in dealing with older adults with physical or cognitive impairments. Effective communication, specialised knowledge, and a commitment to support are essential skills for sex care service providers.

The public discourse in the Netherlands surrounding sex care services often debates whether these services constitute prostitution or healthcare. This ambiguity is exacerbated by the differing legal statuses of various Dutch sex care organisations, with some considered care organisations and others regarded as sex work providers. Despite this, the costs of sex care work are not covered by the healthcare system, although most sex care workers view their work as complementary care (Berkelmans, 2021). Regardless of their official status, sex care workers enhance the sexual, mental and physical health of ageing clients. They address the intimate needs arising from disabilities and impairments, contributing to the overall well-being of these residents.

Practical steps in implementing sex care services in Dutch nursing homes

When nursing homes meet the requirements of providing an open-minded and supportive environment through PCC, sexuality training, sexuality guidelines and employing a sexologist, the support of individual residents will naturally follow. The next subsection of the chapter discusses how sex care workers address individual residents' sexual needs.

Before addressing this, it is essential to consider the issues of financial cost and consent, particularly pertinent when working with older adults with (severe) cognitive impairments. Engaging a sex care worker incurs costs. There are several methods for covering these expenses: some residents use their own funds, others receive financial support from family members, and in rare cases, the local government subsidises the costs. As previously discussed, the socio-economic status of individuals in nursing home care varies. Despite this variation, all residents receive the same level of service within the nursing homes. However, the expenses for sex care workers must be paid by the individual resident, potentially leading to disparities in the frequency of visits. It is interesting to note that the primary barrier for older adults accessing sex care services is not financial constraints. Instead, it often stems from the reluctance of residents who are not in charge of their own money to request funds from family members, as they do not want their families to know about their desire to hire a sex care worker.

Consent in older adults with cognitive impairment is a complex issue. Until recently, there were no universal criteria to determine sexual consent for individuals with cognitive impairment, leaving nursing home care staff and families to assess and determine sexual consent capacity (Huitema-Nuijens, 2022). The sexual consent potential model developed by Huitema and Syme (2023) could be instrumental in supporting care teams to assess and determine sexual consent, thereby addressing this critical issue.

Involving sex care workers is not the first step that is taken when a resident expresses an intimate or sexual need. Instead, there is an elaborate process to determine the resident's actual needs and find the right solutions or care to fulfill those needs. When sex care services are the most suitable way to care for a resident's needs, sex care organisations provide a professional intake and selection procedure to establish if their sex care services are the correct fit (see Figure 9.1).

Residents without cognitive impairment, as potential clients, are able to contact the sex care organisation themselves. In order to involve sex care services the resident needs to fill out an online contact form or complete a phone consultation in which an employee of the sex care service organisation will explain the intake procedure and possibilities. Residents or their supervisors can then ask questions and decide whether the service is a good option. After this decision, the sex care service organisation can ask for information about the resident's background and physical disability and/or cognitive impairment.

Residents with cognitive impairments can get support from sex care service providers, after sexual consent has been determined. When the multidisciplinary care team, mostly in consultation with the legal representative, has decided that the resident is able to consent with regard to involving sex care services, the care team, the caretaker, or the family will likely be needed to support the call to the sex care organisation to set up the service. With the help of a formal direct caregiver or psychologist/sexologist, the residents' needs will be discussed with the sex care organisation. In addition, the spouse or legal representative is informed with the resident's consent.

Figure 9.1: Flow-chart of intake process

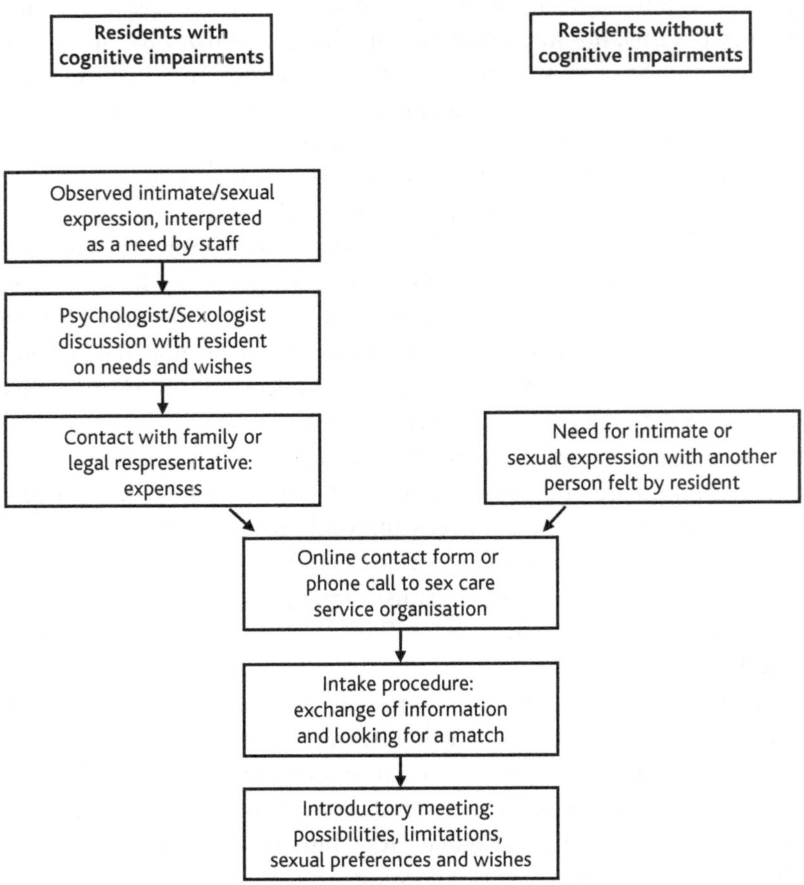

Based on the information provided, the sex care organisation matches a sex care worker to the client. Although the sex care organisation finds a sex care service provider to match the resident's needs, the resident cannot choose specific physical attributes or the age of the sex care service provider. Whereas in regular sex work, a client can choose a sex worker with a specific appearance, nursing home residents who receive services from a sex care organisation cannot. Rather, residents can mainly make requests concerning their sexual orientation and specific sexual preferences. However, specific or more extreme sexual preferences cannot always be met, as sex care service providers are free to set their own boundaries for what services they provide.

If possible, the initial contact between the resident and the sex care worker occurs via telephone, during which they can arrange an introductory meeting at a mutually agreed location and time. This meeting often takes place within the nursing home and aims to establish a rapport, as sex care workers prioritise building relationships with their clients. Residents with physical limitations may choose to have a trusted person present during the meeting, while those with severe cognitive impairments must have a supervisor, such as a direct caregiver or legal representative, in attendance. The first part of the introductory meeting focuses on outlining the possibilities and limitations of both the resident and the sex care worker. The second part addresses the resident's sexual needs for the first time, during which the supervisor may be asked to leave the room. As emphasised by Koenders (2021), 'We [sex care workers] are focused on the well-being of the client'.

All intimate and sexual wishes and needs can be addressed in these meetings. The majority of clients for sex care workers are men, with some requesting male sex care workers. This predominance of male clients may reflect societal constructs and norms that influence how men and women perceive and express their sexual needs and desires. Men, perhaps due to societal encouragement of sexual expression and fewer stigmas associated with seeking sexual services, may be more likely to utilise these services. Conversely, women might experience greater societal barriers and stigmas, resulting in their underrepresentation among sex care clients. Among the small percentage of female clients, approximately half prefer female sex care workers. This preference highlights the importance of personal comfort and safety in these interactions, further illustrating the nuanced nature of sexual needs and preferences among residents in LTC facilities.

> As a male sex worker, I visit male clients through the SAR. Such a visit is for them that extra bit that they do not receive from anyone else. Some seek an intense sexual experience. Others like to talk and experience intimacy. It is wonderful to experience how a client enjoys the touch that is so different from washing, dressing, and medical care. (SAR, n.d.)

After the introductory meeting with the sex care service provider, the resident and supervisor can make an appointment with them for a follow-up visit. The content of the visit is tailored to the sexual and intimate wishes of the client and lasts 1 hour. If residents need extra assistance – such as help getting in and out of bed and getting dressed – the sex care organisation usually asks the formal caregivers to do this, as they know how best to provide this kind of care for each specific resident. However, the sex care service provider performs all sex-related care work. After the sexual experience, hygienic care is completed by the sex care service provider, so that formal caregivers are not confronted with anything that happened during the visit.

Benefits of sex care services

Sex care services are increasingly recognised for their positive impact in the Netherlands, contributing to decreased loneliness and frustration among residents while enhancing their overall happiness (Nwanazia, 2018). Despite the current lack of comprehensive scientific research on the effects of these services, numerous and widespread examples of positive experiences attest to their benefits. The advantages of sex care services extend beyond physical well-being, encompassing psychological benefits for both residents and nursing staff.

One client described the transformative impact of these services, stating, 'My life makes sense again' (SAR, n.d.). Sex care providers strive to establish genuine connections with residents, offering support to those with physical disabilities and/or cognitive impairments. Hans, a sex care provider who exclusively works with men, emphasised the importance of 'compassion without feeling pity' (Smit, 2021). This empathetic approach, treating clients as equals and avoiding condescension, has shown to be particularly beneficial for the clients. Another client highlighted the boost in social confidence, stating, '*I experience more self-confidence when making social contacts*' (SAR, n.d.).

The following examples, drawn from the author's experience as a sexologist in LTC, illustrate the impact of sex care services. For privacy, the names of all residents have been changed.

Mr D, a 76-year-old man living in a semi-independent LTC facility, needed assistance with personal hygiene, medication management and meals. A nurse requested my help with a 'delicate' matter concerning Mr D's desire for intimacy. During our discussion, Mr D expressed his longing for intimate contact. After reviewing the available options, procedures and practicalities, Mr D became excited about the prospect of a sex care worker visiting him. Fortunately, his pension could cover the cost. However, privacy was a significant concern, as the facility housed about 80 residents who were prone to gossip. To address this, we opted for a sex care service organisation experienced in healthcare settings, ensuring discreet visits. This arrangement proved ideal. Months later, Mr D was noticeably happier, more outgoing, and felt 'more alive'. This case demonstrates the improvement in quality of life facilitated by experienced sex care workers. Enhanced resident behaviour and mood positively impacts nursing home staff as well, who find it rewarding to care for happy and healthy residents. Family members, when involved, also appreciate the visible changes in their loved ones, often expressing gratitude to the nursing home.

In some cases, residents had already engaged with sex care workers before their admission to a nursing home. Such arrangements are often overlooked during the admission process. For instance, Mr A, who has Alzheimer's disease, exhibited sexually inappropriate behaviour shortly after his admission. Upon discussing this with Mr A's daughter, the nursing staff learned that he had previously received bi-monthly visits from a sex care worker. The team decided to reinstate these visits after consulting with the daughter about logistics, including finances and hygiene. This decision led to a significant improvement in Mr A's behaviour; he became calmer, more approachable and his inappropriate actions ceased. When his dementia progressed to the point where he could no longer understand the intentions of the sex care provider, the visits were discontinued without negatively affecting his behaviour. This case highlights the necessity of addressing residents' sexual expression to prevent disruptive behaviours and avoid unnecessary medical interventions.

The physical benefits of sex care services extend beyond mere sexual satisfaction, as illustrated by Mrs F's case. Mrs F, a resident with continuous muscle spasms, experienced difficulties with eating, drinking and sleeping. Medication was only partially effective. After a staff training session on sexuality, a nurse inquired about Mrs F's intimacy needs. She welcomed the discussion and embraced the idea of sex care services, given her difficulty handling sex toys due to her spasms. Following the initial visits from a sex care worker, Mrs F's muscle spasms decreased, her sleep improved, and her overall mood brightened, leading to a reduction in her medication. This case underscores the holistic benefits of sex care services, encompassing both physical and psychological well-being.

Conclusion

Resexualisation is a necessity for ageing nursing home residents. Their disabilities and impairments make them highly dependent on their environment, primarily direct and formal caregivers, to address these crucial aspects of life. Although scientific literature on this topic is scarce, the intimate and sexual needs in ageing nursing home residents are gradually being acknowledged in line with the evolution of the PCC paradigm. Policy and staff training on sexuality are increasingly present in Dutch nursing homes, with some nursing homes even including brochures that discuss sexuality upon admission to encourage normalisation. Moreover, the employment of (part-time) sexologists in nursing homes is increasingly encouraging the attention for older adult resexualisation, and the maintenance of an intimate and sexual life during illness and becoming care dependent. They are advocates for this goal as they perform, next to their client-specific work, informative, educational and normalisation work on a national scale.

As demonstrated in this chapter, facilitating access to sex care services can be beneficial for residents. However, it is not a one-size-fits-all solution. Requests pertaining to a resident's sexual needs are highly personal and require a customised approach tailored to the needs of the specific individual. Including these services in nursing home settings is delicate, as not every resident, family member or staff member is willing to discuss this openly (Nwanazia, 2018). Therefore, it is paramount to be respectful to everyone involved and ensure comprehensive staff training.

Sex care services offer more than just sexual satisfaction; they contribute significantly to the quality of life of residents. They foster a sense of belonging and enable residents to communicate on a more deeply intimate level. The experience and expertise of modern sex care workers, many of whom have a background in care professions, allow them to take extra steps in addressing the needs of residents with disabilities or impairments. In a healthcare system that prioritises QoL, the involvement of sex care services is a natural choice for some residents. Beyond the personal benefits for residents, care staff also report positive behavioural changes, including decreased aggression and inappropriate sexual behaviour. Additionally, the professional nature of the practical arrangements often surpasses the expectations of care staff.

Although sex work is legal and regulated in the Netherlands, providing residents with sex care services within a nursing home setting remains uncommon. However, these services enable residents to experience intimacy and sexuality in ways that they want and need. Open discussions about sexuality, viewing it as a normal part of life rather than a problem or unsettling, are necessary and can lead to the increased implementation of sex care services. With this chapter, we aim to destigmatise sex care and inform an international audience about the possibilities of sex care services in Dutch nursing homes.

A literature search on sex workers and people with disabilities and impairments reveals a scarcity of research on this topic. A more specific search on sex workers or sex care services within long-term ageing care resulted in only one publication, from Henrickson et al (2022). This original research from New Zealand investigated care home residents' access to sex workers. The motivation for the study arose from care staff privately admitting during a conference on sexuality in residential care that their facility offered access to sex workers. The researchers became interested in how widespread access to sex workers was in New Zealand, driven by the fear among care staff of being shunned or shamed for providing such access. This brave, first publication shows more work needs to be done to normalise and destigmatise the topic.

Finally, further research is necessary to fully understand the impact and benefits of sex care services in nursing homes. Comprehensive sexuality policies, extensive staff training, and policy changes are essential to effectively resexualise the environment, supporting the individual intimacy needs of residents. Developing staff awareness and sensitivity to these issues, as well as ensuring an environment that respects bodily autonomy and personal choices, are crucial steps in fostering a holistic approach to late-life sexuality. Encouraging open discussions and providing tailored solutions can significantly enhance the QoL for nursing home residents, making intimacy and sexuality a respected and integral part of their care.

Note

1 The term resident is generally used when referring to older individuals residing in nursing home care as the focus is on creating a home, their wellbeing and their agency.

References

Baltes, P.B. and Baltes, M.M. (1990) Psychological perspectives on successful aging: the model of selective optimization with compensation, in P.B. Baltes and M.M. Baltes (eds) *Successful Aging: Perspectives from the Behavioral Sciences*, Cambridge University Press, pp 1–34.

Bauer, M., Fetherstonhaugh, D., Tarzia, L., Nay, R., Wellman, D. and Beattie, E. (2013) 'I always look under the bed for a man': needs and barriers to the expression of sexuality in residential aged care: the views of residents with and without dementia, *Psychology & Sexuality*, 4(3): 296–309.

Berkelmans, L. (2021) Interview on sex care services in Dutch nursing homes [Skype], 17 June.

Chen, Y.H., Jones, C. and Osborne, D. (2017) Exploratory study of Australian aged care staff knowledge and attitudes of later life sexuality, *Australasian Journal of Ageing*, 36: E35–8.

Di Napoli, E.A., Breland, G.L. and Allen, R.S. (2013) Staff knowledge and perceptions of sexuality and dementia of older adults in nursing homes, *Journal of Aging and Health*, 25(7): 1087–105.

Doll, G.M. (2013) Sexuality in nursing homes: practice and policy, *Journal of Gerontological Nursing*, 39(7): 30–7.

Fazio, S., Pace, D., Flinner, J. and Kallmyer, B. (2018) The fundamentals of person-centered care for individuals with dementia, *Gerontologist*, 58(Suppl 1): S10–19.

Henrickson, M., Cook, C.M., MacDonald, S., Atefi, N., & Schouten, V. (2022). Not in the Brochure: *Porneia* and Residential Aged Care. *Sexuality Research and Social Policy*, 19: 588–598.

Huitema-Nuijens, N.N.M. (2022) *The Hidden Expiration Date on Consent: A Delphi Study to Establish Determinants of Sexual Consent in Aging People with Dementia* (publication No. 29207309), Doctoral dissertation, California Institute of Integral Studies, ProQuest Dissertations Publishing.

Huitema, N.N.M. and Syme, M.L. (2023) The sexual consent potential model, *Generations Journal*, 46(4) [online], Available from: https://generations.asaging.org/sexual-consent-potential-model

Koenders, J. (2021) Interview on sex care services in Dutch nursing homes [Skype], 18 June.

Koren, M.J. (2010) Person-centered care for nursing home residents: the culture-change movement, *Health Affairs (Millwood)*, 29(2): 312–17.

Kuyper, L., Verbeek-Oudijk, D. and van Campen, C. (2018) *Jezelf Zijn in het Verpleeghuis [Being Yourself in the Nursing Home]*, Sociaal Cultureel Planbureau.

Mahieu, L. and Gastmans, C. (2015) Older residents' perspectives on aged sexuality in institutionalised elderly care: a systematic literature review, *International Journal of Nursing Studies*, 52(12): 1891–905.

Mahieu, L., Dierckx de Casterlé, B., Acke, J., Vandermarliere, H., Van Elssen, K., Fieuws, S. and Gastmans, C. (2016) Nurses' knowledge and attitudes toward aged sexuality in Flemish nursing homes, *Nursing Ethics*, 23(6): 605–23.

McCormack, B. (2004) Person-centredness in gerontological nursing: an overview of the literature, *Journal of Clinical Nursing*, 13(3a): 31–8.

Nwanazia, C. (2018) Sex care in the Netherlands: helping the disabled find intimacy, *DutchReview* [online], Available at: https://dutchreview.com/culture/relationships/sex-care-in-the-netherlands-helping-the-disabled-find-intimacy/.

Roelofs, T.S.M., Luijkx, K.G. and Embregts, P.J.C.M. (2015) Intimacy and sexuality of nursing home residents with dementia: a systematic review, *International Psychogeriatrics*, 27(3): 367–84.

Roelofs, T.S., Luijkx, K.G. and Embregts, P.J. (2019) Love, intimacy and sexuality in residential Dementia care: a spousal perspective, *Dementia*, 18(3): 936–50.

Roelofs, T.S.M., Luijkx, K.G. and Embregts, P.J.C.M. (2021) Love, intimacy and sexuality in residential dementia care: a client perspective, *Clinical Gerontology*, 44(3): 288–98.

Sion, K.Y.J., Verbeek, H., de Boer, B., Zwakhalen, S.M.G., Odekerken-Schroder, G., Schols, J.M.G.A. and Hamers, J.P.H. (2020) How to assess experienced quality of care in nursing homes from the client's perspective: results of a qualitative study, *BMC Geriatrics*, 20(1), DOI:10.1186/s12877-020-1466-7

Smit, N. (2021) Gehandicapten willen ook gewoon seks; gesprek met hans [Disabled people also just want to have sex; conversation with hand], Podcast De StellingCast, 20 May [online], Available from: https://www.vgn.nl/podcast-de-stellingcast

Stichting Alternatieve Relatiebemiddeling [Alternative Relationship Mediation Foundation] (SAR) (n.d.) Each person has need for warmth and intimacy [online], Available from: https://www.stichtingsar.nl/index.html

Syme, M.L. (2014) The evolving concept of older adult sexual behavior and its benefits, *Generations: Journal of American Society on Aging*, 38(1): 35–41.

Thys, K., Mahieu, L., Cavolo, A., Hensen, C., Dierckx de Casterle, B. and Gastmans C. (2019) Nurses' experiences and reactions towards intimacy and sexuality expressions by nursing home residents: a qualitative study, *Journal of Clinical Nursing*, 28(5–6): 836–49.

Tzeng, Y.-L., Lin, L.-C., Shyr, Y.-I.L. and Wen, J.-K. (2009) Sexual behaviour of institutionalised residents with dementia: a qualitative study, *Journal of Clinical Nursing*, 18(7): 991–1001.

Vandrevala, T., Chrysanthaki, T. and Ogundipe, E. (2017) 'Behind closed doors with open minds?': A qualitative study exploring nursing home staff's narratives towards their roles and duties within the context of sexuality in dementia, *International Journal of Nursing Studies*, 74: 112–19.

Waterschoot, K., Roelofs, T.S.M., van Boekel, L.C. and Luijkx, K.G. (2022) Care staff's sense-making of intimate and sexual expressions of people with dementia in Dutch nursing homes, *Clinical Gerontologist*, 45(4): 833–43.

Wet Langdurige Zorg [WLZ] (2024) *Long-term Care Act* [online], Available from: https://wetten.overheid.nl/BWBR0035917/2024-07-01.

10

Resexualising older disabled people's sexual and intimate lives: an outline, framework and research agenda

Susan Gillen and Paul Reynolds

In Gillen and Reynolds (2021a, b – the second volume of this book series) we explored the desexualisation of older disabled people's sexual and intimate lives, not as a natural feature of ageing and disability, but as a constructed interweaving of pathological and prejudicial discourses characterising sex, age and disability. These discourses stretch across both physical and intellectual disability, involving both common constraints and particular forms reflecting the diversity and plurality of impairments and disabling processes and structures. We argued that due to the prevalence and embeddedness of desexualisation in society, which impedes, among other things, the capacity of sexual agents to have sexual and intimate agency represented positively in the public sphere, a revolutionary approach to care, support and enabling is required if we are to reconceive current constraints into contingencies and opportunities.

In this chapter, as a way of exploring potentially creative avenues for resexualisation, and of ultimately bolstering the view of the older disabled as full(er) social citizens, we outline and focus on examples of empirical evidence related to three broad areas: policy and practice, sex care and technology. We argue that a person centred care (PCC) approach to sexual expression is needed in order to promote autonomy and choice, to appreciate both values and preferences – and we can include here intimate and sexual preferences – and where the guiding principle for such an approach should be 'beneficence rather than non-maleficence'. In other words, the ability to exercise sexual rights should be taken for granted until proven otherwise' (Villar, 2019: 164). That said, no matter how positive the examples may be, or their potential is to enable and empower the older disabled, an awareness throughout is crucial of how sexual agency is connected to wider social, economic and cultural inequalities, which in turn impacts the capacity of an individual to exercise their wishes. Shakespeare (1996), for example, emphasised how class is a powerful determinant of the disability experience; similarly Walker and Foster (2006) highlight the enduring relationship between social class and ageing. It is fundamental then to consider that older people experience their sexual and intimate relations as intersectional agents. While our focus in this chapter is primarily on the intersections of age and disability, there must be recognition that these relationships are influenced by other identarian differences such as gender, ethnicity, sexuality and class (and, at times, their dynamic nature) which results in different experiences of sexual quality of life. We end the chapter with a suggested framework for future research that takes into account the fundamental nature of resexualisation and the importance of agency for sexual equity of the older disabled.

Policy and practice

The 'wheels of change' in relation to policy can be slow to turn, with a tendency for incremental rather than dynamic transformations, and while policy enactment in and of itself is not a guarantee for changes in practice, and needs in particular to recognise and account for the professional, organisational and social contexts for the policy implementation (see, for example, Watt et al, 2005), policy, it is argued, remains a fundamental determinant, and indeed requirement, in the care, support and enabling for many older people with disabilities in relation to sexual expression (see, for example, Lester et al, 2016; Villar et al, 2017). Laws and policies can be an enabler or disabler:

> Laws and policies matter because they set rules and frameworks for people's conduct in society and for programmatic interventions. They can contribute to or obstruct the development of programmatic and service delivery interventions on sexual health, deter or support people's experience of sexual pleasure, and enable or disable people to seek and receive the information they require to protect their sexual health and exercise their sexual rights. (Gruskin et al, 2019: 32)

These points are particularly relevant to older disabled people whose sexual health and rights are often undermined and controlled through policies and practices that lead to the inaccessibility of sexuality and sexual health information/services, or the presumption that the ageing process changes people's needs (see Kismödi et al, 2015; Harnett and Jönson, 2017, cited in Larsson and Jönson, 2018).

However, it is often the lack of specific, clear or relevant policy (Evans et al, 2009; Lester et al, 2016; McAuliffe et al, 2020; Charitou et al, 2021), or issues related to its implementation (English and Tickle, 2018), that are highlighted as barriers to the expression of sexuality and intimacy. The relationship between policy and practice is complex and embodies a quandary; while the aim of policy is to solve problems, the policy authors, often the government, are not usually those with the solutions – the problem solvers are those with the problem, but they may lack agency or other means to enact solutions. This lack of agency has been highlighted, particularly, in care home settings. For example, Bahner's (2019) policy analysis and qualitative research across four countries (the UK, Australia, Sweden and the Netherlands) highlighted how the relationship between policy and practice in care settings is not straightforward and how there is a 'multitude of intersectional aspects at play and they largely mirror broadly structural inequalities in society, with the added dimensions of ableism and disablism in the mix' (p 211). Bahner's work, nevertheless, highlights the potential for policy to support the development of sexual support services.

As with Bahner's work, there appears to be variability in policy approaches to support disabled people in expressing their sexuality (Bahner, 2019: 98). While it is recognised that there is a need for policies and practices which promote sexual citizenship (see, for example, Richardson, 2000; Lester et al, 2016; Villar et al, 2017) such policies are few and far between. Nevertheless there are examples, globally, of policy to support sexual expression that we can draw on. In the UK, the Royal College of Nursing (2022) have developed guidance to support training and best practice for care workers and professionals. Furthermore, the Care Quality Commission (CQC) have provided guidelines for adult social care (ASC) for expressing sexuality; their 2019 report provides a review of sexual safety and the support of people's sexuality in ASC and is based on developing an empowering organisational culture based on PCC principles. It is interesting to note here that the emphasis is first placed 'on safety' rather than 'on support' despite the CQC's (2020: 6) own review of sexual safety in adult social care which notes that, in relation to sexual abuse incidents, 'These sexual incidents are not common. Sexual incidents made up around 3% of the total notifications of abuse or alleged abuse we received in our review period.'

Nevertheless, Charitou et al (2021) in their systematic review of qualitative research into the support for 'Adults with Intellectual Disabilities with Relationships and Sex' are hopeful that such developments can 'gradually lead to a change in culture within services and the elimination of disempowering and restrictive views' (2021: 141).

There are several practical ways to implement such policy and guidelines into practice, and facilitate sexual expression, via access to sexual health information, products and services, and with staff who are trained to facilitate the sexual health needs of residents. These practicalities do not just relate to care homes but to private homes, too. A phenomenological study by Linton and Williams (2019) in the United States of America (US) aimed at understanding the perspective of social workers in supporting intimate couples where at least one was older with a disability, concluded that whether clients were supported in their homes or in institutions, two aspects of life were very important to ensuring intimate and sex relationships: privacy and beds. Indeed this is supported by Roelofs et al's (2021) recent qualitative research looking at the perspective of residents with dementia and their spouses with regard to love, intimacy, and sexuality, who found barriers to sexual expression in the form of a lack of double beds: 'Couple FG shared that they sleep in two single beds, which are put together in the same bedroom. The male spouse said that a double bed would not fit in their bedroom' (2021: 292).

There was also an absence of privacy:

> (Referring to) the experience of couple EF, who were sexually active in the RCF. They did discuss the absence of a feeling of privacy. This absence of privacy persisted despite the 'do not disturb' sign they used for the bedroom. The female spouse explained that it is still sometimes difficult for her and her husband to feel comfortable at the RCF, because 'It is not exactly like home.' She for example, only feels comfortable taking her top off, but does not feel comfortable enough to take more clothes off. (2021: 292–3)

Further, in research by Rahn et al (2020: 57) which looked at baby boomers' attitudes to maintaining sexual and intimate relationships in residential care, participants highlighted the need for access to qualified sexual health professionals, lubricants, condoms, sex toys and erotic material and 'visual privacy … private space and protected communication' in order to promote autonomy, self respect and dignity.

> It would be important to be able to obtain products (eg lubricants etc) without the embarrassment of having to ask family etc. (MR113 cited in Rahn et al, 2020: 55)

> People may not be able to get out to a pharmacy or they may not have the privacy they need to speak about intimate issues to their GP [general practitioner] so they would need products and information on site. (FR29 cited in Rahn et al, 2020: 55)

Other ways to facilitate the implementation of policy changes is to support the staff to develop a PCC approach; for example, the use of PCC thinking tools, training or organisational support (see, for example, Skills for Care, 2020; Helen Anderson Associates, 2021). Examples of such policy approaches/tools do exist. In Australia, for example, they have developed a 'Sexuality Assessment Tool (SexAT)', based on both the available literature and verified by interviews with care staff, residents and families (Bauer et al,

2014). It provides a gap analysis style and scoring system to assist with policy development within the long-term care settings and its aim is to support the normalisation of sexuality, enhance policy/practice/training and monitor initiatives. The tool is wide ranging and focuses on a number of 'broad areas' including facility policies (ranging from the provision of 'do not disturb' signs, the incorporation of sexuality into assessment and care planning, through to access to sex workers, if legal); information and support (for example, provision of sexual aids, condoms and audio-visual aids); the environment (such as the availability of double beds) and staff training/expertise. Another example that is available to support healthcare professionals is the PLISSIT (Permission, Limited Information, Specific Suggestions and Intensive Therapy) model originally developed by a psychologist in 1976 for the treatment of sexual issues, which is available to facilitate discussion regarding sexual well-being needs (Freak-Poli, 2020).

Alternatively, the extended Ex-PLISSIT model which, among other things, sees 'permission-giving' as the core feature of all stages (Taylor and Davis, 2007). In the UK an interactive training resource to engage and meet the sexuality and intimacy needs of care home residents has been developed (Horne et al, 2022) in response to the training needs identified by care home staff and in Vancouver, Canada they have developed a policy for Supporting Sexual Health and Intimacy in Care Facilities (Vancouver Coastal Health Authority, 2013) which provides guidelines to help individual care providers to, in turn, develop their own guidelines. This covers a range of areas from autonomy for sexual expression, responsibilities for care givers, decision making, consent/capability, risk assessment, through to information and assistance with sexual expression, privacy and confidentiality; all of which is underpinned by staff training. These guidelines were developed as a result of research consisting of a focus group (held over 2 days) of health providers, persons with disabilities, older adults, representatives from advocacy groups and experts in healthcare ethics and law, plus an international literature and policy review, together with personal communications with experts in a range of fields from ethics, sexual health and the law (Everett et al, 2010).

An exemplar, according to Bentrott and Margrett (2017), of service provision that has proactively established appropriate policies, is the Hebrew Home at Riverdale, New York (2017) which provides a range of services for older people including those with dementia. This organisation, taking a PCC approach, has an established sexual expression policy and sexually relevant materials to support the residents, their families and the staff in understanding residents' rights to remain sexually expressive (Bentrott-Margrett, 2017).

Finally, in this section, an interesting proposal by Hill (2014: 472) which looks at the idea of decision making tools for preserving sexual autonomy, is the completion of a 'sexual power of attorney' and/or advance directives clarifying wishes regarding sexual relationships. Boni-Saenz (2016) who posed the question 'Can one consent to sex in advance?' also considers the benefits of this approach in the context of an ageing population where more people will suffer from cognitive impairments as they age into disability. He argues that such policies present the possibility of a sexual life for those diagnosed with chronic conditions that affect cognition and threaten their legal capacity for decision making. Sexual directives would allow for the person to consent prospectively to sex or, alternatively, empower an agent to make decisions about sex on their behalf. Boni-Saenz suggests there are three main reasons older people may benefit from the development of sexual advance directives: 'They might have an interest in enabling sexually fulfilling lives for their future disabled selves, in preserving important sexual identities or relationships, or in protecting spouses from criminal prosecution for rape' (2016: 4).

While this may be of benefit in all settings, it may be particularly helpful in residential care due to restrictive policies and attitudes to older age sexuality which can threaten their sexual self-determination.

The examples in this section emphasise the dichotomous nature of policy as both being an enabler and disabler of sexual equity for the older disabled. However, even taking into account the emphasis on a PCC approach, they do not explicitly stress the need or offer practical examples to consider the multiplicative effect of age and disability with other identarian differences such as gender, ethnicity and class. This is not to say that there is a lack of recognition in the policy arena to use an intersectional lens to avoid the conscious or unconscious oppression of individuals based on such identities; indeed in the UK a recent Department of Health blog (2020) in relation to social work, specifically stresses that an intersectional analysis is 'key for navigating the multiple and complex needs of older people who are (also) members of oppressed groups'.

However, examples of intersectional praxis are few and far between. Similarly, Humphries et al (2023) in their analysis of public health policy in the US, argue that while intersectional approaches have been key in highlighting the 'compounded risks and synergistic disparities experienced by individuals impacted by multiple forces of oppression' (2023: 2) the focus has been mainly theoretical and analytical, with little or no practical application. The need then to develop intersectionality praxis and transformative solutions is argued to be fundamental (Bowleg, 2021).

One such example, to end this section with, is the Intersectionality-Based Policy Analysis (IBPA) framework developed in the US by Hankivsky et al (2014) which, in recognising the negative impacts that policies can have (see, for example, Richardson, 2016), and of the need to integrate values, social justice and equity, uses a structured questioning process when developing policy and practice. Its aim as a policy tool is not only to provide a structure for critical policy analysis, but to do this within different dimensions of policy contexts such as time and place, and furthermore to generate action orientated, transformative policy solutions. While Hankivsky et al (2014) have not focused their work specifically on the older disabled, they have demonstrated in a number of case studies the potential of IBPA to offer transformative policy analysis that can translate intersectionality theory into practical approaches and, thereby, may offer a potential avenue for the resexualisation of the older disabled that recognises them as intersectional agents.

Sex care

While policy developments might be slow to materialise, there are illustrations of the sexual rights for people with disabilities being translated into tangible measures. One such measure, discussed in this section, is the development of special sex services, or referred to here as 'sex care' which can broadly be applied to the roles of sexual therapists, advisers, facilitators and surrogates, and aims to support both partnered and unpartnered (older) adults with disabilities. Of course sex work is not a new phenomenon, and has been proclaimed as the 'oldest profession' (Wotton, 2020) with the sex industry operating in almost all countries throughout the world in one form or another. However, despite the contentious nature of sex work and its links to debates around prostitution (see, for example, Jahnsen and Wagenaar, 2017), it is argued that the last 15 years or so has seen the emergence of new ways of organising and developing policy related to 'sex care' from a disability rights movement perspective (Geymonat, 2019).

One example of this is the Netherlands where the provision of 'sex care' is provided by healthcare professionals (sex care workers) and is aimed specifically at people with severe disabilities, both physical and mental, focusing on physical touch, intimacy and sexual satisfaction (Nwanazia, 2018). Sex care workers, who can be hired for a fee by the client, their family or a health/social professional, are provided by various organisations which Nwanazia refers to as 'erotic service providers'. The overriding aim is to improve the quality of life. As one disabled man said:

> the beauty of sex care in the Netherlands is that you can freely go on a journey to discover your sexuality without feeling shame or guilt. You are a human being just like everyone else and it is your right to live your life to the fullest – disabled or not. (Nwanazia, 2018).

Another example of the acknowledgment of the erotic lives of people with disabilities and the positive implementation of sex care is in Denmark where sex workers are trained to be sexual advisers (seksualvejleder) and facilitators. Kulick and Rydstrom's (2015) ethnographic research, which in fact took place in both Denmark and Sweden, focuses on the sexual and erotic lives of adults with physical or intellectual disabilities who are more likely to depend on others to enable them to explore or experience their sexuality. Their research demonstrates how both countries take different approaches to the caring practices of the sexualities of those with disabilities, with Denmark taking what can be seen as an active engagement, whereas Sweden's approach is that of disabled sexuality being a problem and effectively silencing it. Both approaches, therefore, are underpinned by the cultural attitudes and care giving that either impedes or facilitates the erotic lives of those with disabilities and highlights how ultimately those cultural attitudes also play out in policy and guidelines. Interestingly we see links here between legislation in both countries, where in Denmark sex workers are legalised, while in Sweden they are prohibited, highlighting how political issues of the criminalisation of sex work coincides with approaches to dealing with disabled people's sex lives.

Other service examples are those that are provided in the form of collaborations, either between different organisations which offer sexual services, such as the European Platform for Sexual Assistance for people with disabilities (EPSEAS, 2021) who currently have partners in Switzerland, Spain, Belgium, Italy, Czech Republic, Netherlands and France, or those that offer direct connections between disabled people and sex workers such as Touching Base in Australia (2021) or TLC (2021) in the UK.

Another form of 'sex care' is sexual surrogacy; this is not a new phenomenon, developed as a form of sexual therapy in the 1960s, it remains as contentious today as it did back then. The most common framework enacted is that of a therapist-client-surrogate triangulated model where, based on a sexual therapist's recommendations given an individual's experience of sexual issues, the individual may engage with a paid sex worker, or surrogate, to help them address their issues (Shapiro, 2017). However, a trained sex worker/surrogate may also work/advertise their services independently. Paid sexual services are not just about stimulation of the genitals – they are wide-ranging and vary in relation to the type of service, location and price. The aim is to provide a mutually consenting service for clients. Wotton (2016b cited in Wotton, 2020) identified over 20 different types of services that sex workers provided to their clients with disability including: 'hand relief (masturbation), oral sex, vaginal sex, anal sex, fantasies, roleplays, nude body slides, nude massage, striptease, Bondage, Discipline, Sadism and Masochism (BDSM), strap-on services (pegging), use of vibrators and Spanish ("tit fucking")' (2020: 435).

Shapiro (2017: 134) argues that 'surrogacy … is about helping individuals discover their inherent erotic natures and acquire the tools they need to manifest their erotic natures with themselves and their partners'. Shapiro, a trained sex surrogate in the US, who, himself, has a disability, however, cautions the role of sex surrogacy, itself, furthering stereotypes of the able-bodied sexual surrogate supporting the needy disabled person: 'I tire of the endless image of the benevolent able-bodied surrogate "helping" the socially isolated disabled man. There needs to be a greater understanding and awareness of disabled people as sexual beings beyond the objectification of disabled people as receivers of sexual services' (2017: 137).

Shapiro highlights the significance of the medical gaze of the disabled – and we can add to this, the older – body. For Shapiro, not only should there be more access to training for surrogates and to the surrogates themselves for disabled people, but for those surrogate services to be provided by a disabled person: 'If there is such a thing as "sexual leadership," disabled people must pursue it if we are ever to overcome the stereotypes of surrogacy' (2017: 137).

While these examples suggest there is an increasing recognition of the sexual rights of the disabled person, and we can add to this the older person, there are in fact few internationally recognised organisations that support clients with disability to engage with sex workers, although there are examples in the Netherlands, Denmark, UK, Switzerland and Australia, with training organisations established in South Africa, the Czech Republic and Germany (see Wotton, 2020). Wotton, once a sex worker herself for over 26 years, and based on her own research, explored a range of models of paid sexual services aimed at people with disabilities, including sex work, surrogacy, sexual assistants, masturbation services and training providers. Recognising the complexity of such services, including the lack of education, awareness, policies, funding, plus moral and ethical debates, her aim ultimately was to build awareness of the current practices to support positive legislative change globally – arguing this will be of benefit to the different disability and ageing sectors when considering how best to support their clients' needs and sexual expression. Wotton can be argued to take a PCC approach as she argues for choice and autonomy for all:

> While it should always remain an individual decision to seek out sexual services, or not, ultimately the fundamental issue is about choice and respecting the person's autonomy, with no difference in this equation as a result of a person's disability. While it's imperative to emphasise that this should never be the only 'go-to' option for people with disability, it should not be dismissed either. Rather, it should be regarded as just one of many options people with disability should be able to choose from, as with anyone else in society. (Wotton, 2020: 445)

Notwithstanding the possibilities highlighted in this section in relation to the sexual rights of the older disabled, Wooton's comments here regarding the complexities of sexual service, particularly in relation to access, funding, choice and autonomy, remind us of the need to explore issues through an intersectional lens. Using the ability to pay for sex care services as an example, it is fair to say that not all older people or all disabled people would be disadvantaged in this regard; certainly if we intersect disability or age with class relations, it is clear that those of a higher class may command significant resources. Nevertheless, poverty is argued to be a particular risk for both the disabled (Schwendel, 2020) and older people (United Nations, 2022). So, too, older women, suffer from higher levels of poverty than older men (United Nations, 2022). Thus we need to be aware of the multidimensional aspects of privilege and disadvantage to consider how inequalities, discrimination and oppression based on identarian differences interact. In terms of the inability to pay or access sex care, it follows that for some, if the services are not provided free by the state or organisations, this may serve to be a significant barrier to sexual equity.

Technology

As highlighted in the second volume of this book series (Gillen and Reynolds, 2021a, b), while it is the case that the burden and convergence of chronic disease and disability in later life impacts on older people's sexual health and well-being (Lee et al, 2016; Erens et al, 2019), research by Freak-Poli (2020) suggests that partner availability may be the greatest barrier to being sexually active in older age. In her re-analysis of data from a study of 2,374 Dutch older adults, she observed that older partnered adults were 15 times more likely than unpartnered older adults to engage in sexual activity. This section focuses on two areas that offer potential technological opportunities for the disabled older adult to address the problem of a lack of a partner: sex robots and internet dating.

Sex robots

Sex robots, or sexbots, are anthropomorphic robotic dolls with a 'human like appearance, movement and behaviour designed to interact with people in erotic and romantic ways … with capabilities ranging from simple verbal responses, to physical movements, to more advanced artificial intelligence' (Gersen, 2019 cited in Jecker, 2020: 26). They typically have different embodiments, have animatronic heads and faces that move, arms and genitals for sex-related tasks, realistic silicone skin and, unlike sex dolls, can include human cues such as such as voice or gaze (Fosch-Villaronga and Poulsen, 2021). They are designed to facilitate interactive experiences that simulate being with a 'live and present human being' and as such are distinct from sex toys.

The use of sex robots has mixed reactions in terms of their use ethically (see, for example, Gersen, 2019; Earp and Grunt-Mejer, 2021) and their impact – both positive or negative – is, as yet, unknown (Fosch-Villaraonga and Poulsen, 2021). Some argue that sex robots might 'not be enough' in terms of a satisfactory replacement for human sexual interaction (Boni-Saenz, 2021). Furthermore, technology often brings problems as well as solutions; for example, there is a danger they might reinforce existing biases (such as objectification of women) (see Richardson, 2015) and in relation to care in particular, there is a danger of the 'dehumanisation of care'. Nevertheless, even though they may not be the ideal method of sexual interaction, they may have a part to play, in particular, with older age disability (Boni-Saenz, 2021). Koumpis and Gees (2020), whose research into healthy ageing and well-being looked at robots as a way of help older people to cope with isolation and loneliness, argued that if there is the 'potential to offer comfort to anyone, irrespective of age, abilities or disabilities and any other characteristics, it is something that we should all consider in a positive way, if not a welcome one' (2020: 230).

Also, Fosch-Villaraonga and Poulsen (2021) consider the notion of sex robots being a step towards empowering people with disabilities to exercise their sexual rights, arguing that they can be designed to support the sexual, emotional and educational needs for people with disabilities:

> As a tool, sex robots could help provide a safe environment for persons with disabilities to explore sexuality. Some sex robots, such as Rocky or Roxxxy, can perform simple sexual movements, i.e., moving back and forth from the user rather than requiring them to move. This function could be useful for those with physical disabilities as it affords the user the ability to use a sex robot without high physical cost. Furthermore, sex robots that enable masturbation, such as Gabriel2052 with a robotic arm or a Realdollx model with a massaging function, could cater to a physically disabled user's need. (2021: 4)

Furthermore, Bianchi (2021) suggests that sex robots offer specific benefits to people with cognitive impairments and, in particular for those older people with dementia where issues of consent are paramount, sex robots would provide a way to fulfil sexual needs with issues of consent. Jecker (2020), focusing specifically on older people with disabilities, argues that we should afford access to sex robots to support their ability to express their sexuality. This may serve to address barriers to older age sex, that is, supporting older people with disability or chronic diseases who need assistance to engage in sexual activities (Jecker, 2020) or providing an 'alternative' where partner availability is limited.

However, following the ageist stereotype of the asexual older person, currently the marketing and design of sex robots is focused on the young, able bodied and male client (Jecker, 2020). Nevertheless, the benefits of such a cultural change are argued, from both a utilitarian perspective and capability approaches. Jecker takes the latter approach and suggests that 'the ability to function sexually is linked to central human capabilities' (2020: 28). Arguing that society has a duty to support these capabilities at a minimal threshold, she purports that sex robots are one mechanism for enhancing life narratives by generating counternarratives, by not only affording access to sex robots, but designing them with older people in mind. The assistance of sex robots provides one tool for older people with disability to gain control, autonomy and choice over their sexual lives and thus maintain their sexual health. In terms of care settings, as a minimum, their inclusion could help the recognition of the sexual rights of the users (Fosch-Villaronga and Poulsen, 2021). While the sex robots have raised an ethical debate, and not withstanding earlier points in the previous section about affordability and the need to take use an intersectional analysis, Jecker's position has offered a stimulus for creative thinking about how to support older disabled people's sexual desires.

Internet dating

Internet dating is a relatively new phenomenon, starting in the mid 1990s following the establishment of the 'net', and is a popular way of forming social connections involving sexuality, providing opportunities for 'digital intimacy' (Hategan et al, 2016) and for people to find more potential partners than they are likely to encounter through normal social contacts. While recognising the risks and trust issues related to this form of dating (see, for example, Chen et al, 2020) early research by Couch and Liamputtong (2008) suggests that it 'allows for greater connectivity between people, providing the opportunity for enhanced social and sexual networks' (2008: 277), facilitating networking and communication regardless of mobility limitations. As such, internet dating offers a way to link the sexual practice of older people to social change (Beasley and Holmes, 2016) and is an illustrative example of enabling an escape from the usual social conventions, allowing new possibilities.

Despite research in the field of older people and internet use/dating being limited, with a propensity for a health and safety focus, looking, for example, at STIs (Couch et al, 2011), condom use (Bateson et al, 2012) and the risk of victimisation, and regardless of ageist assumptions about the asexual and technophobic older person, evidence suggests that the number of older people accessing the net is increasing (Malta, 2007; Beasley and Holmes, 2016). Given the predicted size of the older adult demographic, finding a partner online may quickly become the 'norm' for much of this generation:

> For decades, as a group, [the Baby Boomers] have challenged and pushed the limits of … norms; redefining the concepts of family

> and sexual expression (among many others) … we should anticipate increased changes and challenges in other social norms as this huge cohort moves into later life … Their technological competence and relative affluence will increase the potential of the Internet as a source of personal and social expression of sexuality in later life. (Adams et al, 2003, cited in Malta, 2007: 91)

That said, there may be problems with access to using this online technology; as people age either into or with a disability, chronic disease of ageing, including neurocognitive disorders such as dementia can impair daily function and, while online data sites may not discriminate, an inability to master basic IT skills means support may be required. There may be specific issues, also, in relation to older adults within institutional settings, where there is seemingly no data available (Hategan et al, 2016). Nevertheless Malta's (2007) study of 61–85 year olds found that older people were comparatively nimble to becoming intimate, sexually, with those they met online. For example, all, bar one of her participants met their online partners face-to-face, and all engaged in sexual activity the first time they met:

> We couldn't keep our hands off each other when we were first together. (Female: 82 years)

> We knew on first sight that we would end up in bed … Once we had slept together… we both felt it was the most wonderful sex we'd ever experienced – and it still is! Amazing… (Female: 72 years)

Discussions in this section suggest there is potential for technology to support the resexualisation of the older disabled. While the development of sex robots is in its infancy, the internet and social dating sites are not; they are the second most common way that dating couples meet (Cocalis, 2016, cited in Lamphere and Pomykacz, 2022). Significantly, in the UK in 2023 there were 11.1 million online dating users (Statista, 2024), estimated to increase to 12 million in the next 5 years. However, as well as the possibilities that technology offers in this medium to support sexual equity, there are concerns being raised about social inequalities, such as those related to ageism, sexism, homophobia and disability discrimination, being reproduced in online spaces (Lamphere and Pomyacz, 2022). Such inequalities are rooted in discriminating and limiting ideas about age, disability, gender, ethnicity and sexuality. While digital technologies can expand our access to the wider community and thus the opportunity to find potential sexual and intimate partners, how far it can go to achieve sexual equity, it is argued, requires a deeper understanding of both the root causes of inequalities and the intersections of disadvantage, rather than limiting ourselves to a singular or superficial technological solution.

Where we go from here: a framework and research agenda

The previous discussion has prompted us to think about where we go next in terms of research policy and practice. We have emphasised the need for a revolutionary approach to care, support and enabling, in order for the older disabled to have sexual and intimate agency, and focusing on the three broad areas of policy and practice, 'sex care' and technology, we have explored creative avenues for resexualisation, emphasising here the need to develop a PCC approach to sexual expression. Certainly from looking at the examples of empirical evidence discussed there seems scope for optimism.

At the policy level, for instance, while recognising that the prevalence and embeddedness of desexualisation is such that incremental policy change may have a limited and slow impact, there are some excellent examples of good practice highlighted and it is argued that policy remains a fundamental determinant in the promotion of sexual citizenship, where laws and policies can be an enabler. Also, while it is perhaps unlikely, given current policy priorities of the government and policy makers, that the 'wheels of change' will move speedily, there are positive shifts such as the contemporary narrative to care generally being towards a holistic approach, with an emphasis on individualisation, autonomy and self-determination (see, for example, the Health and Social Care Act 2008, Regulations 9 and 14) and the recognition of the need to use an intersectional lens in social work practice; this might suggest a level of optimism in terms of supporting the resexualisation of older people with disabilities. The discussions around 'sex care' also provide optimism, suggesting there is an increasing recognition of the sexual rights of the disabled person, an emergence of new ways of delivering sex care to people with disabilities and an understanding of the need for more agency for the recipients of sexual services.

However, the research also highlights the significance of historical and contemporary environments, where attitudes to sex care is both cultural and political (and, as such, not always positive). And while not highlighted specifically in the research already outlined, consideration of the commercialisation of such 'services' is key; it may, for example, serve to exclude those that cannot afford to 'pay'. The third area of empirical evidence discussed was the use of technology. Sex robots were seen as both empowering and offering potential, yet raised ethical issues – the jury is still out as to their impact; nevertheless it offers us a stimulus for creative thinking, although also raises issues of inequity in terms of access. So, too, internet dating, albeit raising issues of potentially reproducing social inequalities in a digital sphere, on a positive note offers a potential enabler; as Beasley and Holmes (2016) argue, it offers a vehicle to link the sexual practice of older people to social change.

We have stressed in this chapter the need to recognise how sexual agency is connected to wider social, economic and cultural inequalities and to consider that older people experience their sexual and intimate relations as intersectional agents. While there are some clear themes that have emerged through our discussion broadly in terms of future research ideas, such as the need for specific, clear or relevant policy, enabling the 'problem solvers' to develop agency, and the need for more training, it is limiting to focus simply on separate pieces of potential research areas or themes. The very complex and dynamic nature of resexualisation itself lends to the need for a clear framework to support all future research. If we recognise that resexualisation works on three levels: an understanding of the spatial, temporal, representational, cultural and political relations, materialities and discourses by which desexualisation is constructed and sustained; a counterhegemonic strategy that dissembles these factors and pathologies and prejudices, both imposed upon and internalised; and a creative space where the nexus of sex, age and disability can be reconceived to focus on pleasure, intimate expression and productive relations and discursive constructs within changed material conditions, then it follows that this framework needs to take all three into account. Such a framework should by underpinned by recognition of the heterogeneity and intersectionality of sexuality by age, dis/ability, gender, ethnicity and class, consideration of the spatial reality in terms of the historical and environmental context, and take into account the dynamic nature of sexuality; and in so doing should support a research agenda to enable agency and sexual equity for older people who are disabled and for whom ageing brings disability.

References

Bahner, J. (2019) *Sexual Citizenship and Disability: Understanding Sexual Support in Policy, Practice and Theory*, Routledge.

Bateson, D.J., Weisberg, E., McCaffery K.J. and Luscombe, G.M. (2012) When online becomes offline: attitudes to safer sex practices in older and younger women using an australian internet dating service, *Sex Health*, 9(2): 152–9.

Bauer, M., Fetherstonhaugh, D., Tarzia, L., Nay, R. and Beattie, E. (2014) Supporting residents' expression of sexuality: the initial construction of a sexuality assessment tool for residential aged care facilities, *British Medical Council, Geriatrics*, 14: 82, DOI: 10.1186/1471-2318-14-82.

Beasley, C. and Holmes, M. (2016) Internet dating, sexual intimacy and older people, in E. Peel and R. Harding (eds) *Ageing and Sexualities: Interdisciplinary Perspectives*, Routledge, pp 205–22.

Bentrott, M. and Margrett, J. (2017) Adopting a multilevel approach to protecting residents' rights to sexuality in the long-term care environment: policies, staff training, and response strategies, *Sexuality Research and Social Policy*, 14, DOI: 10.1007/s13178-016-0260-y.

Bianchi, A. (2021) Considering sex robots for older adults with cognitive impairments, *Journal of Med Ethics*, 47: 37–8.

Boni-Saenz, A.A. (2016) Sexual advance directives, *Alabama Law Review*, 68(1): 1–47.

Boni-Saenz, A.A. (2021) Are sex robots enough?, *Journal of Medical Ethics*, 47: 35.

Bowleg, L. (2021) Evolving intersectionality within public health: from analysis to action, *American Journal of Public Health*, 111: 88–90.

Care Quality Commission (CQC) (2019) *Relationships and Sexuality in Adult Social Care Services: Guidance for CQC Inspection staff and Registered Adult Social Care Providers*, CQC [online], Available from: https://www.cqc.org.uk/sites/default/files/20190221-Relationships-and-sexuality-in-social-care-PUBLICATION.pdf

CQC (2020) *Promoting Sexual Safety through Empowerment: a Review of Sexual Safety and the Support of People's Sexuality in Adult Social* Care, CQC [online], Available from: https://www.cqc.org.uk/sites/default/files/20200225_sexual_safety_sexuality.pdf

Charitou, M., Quayle, E. and Sutherland, A. (2021) Supporting adults with intellectual disabilities with relationships and sex: a systematic review and thematic synthesis of qualitative research with staff, *Sex and Disability*, 39: 113–46.

Chen, Q., Yuan, Y. Feng, Y. and Archer N. (2020) A decision paradox: benefit vs risk and trust vs distrust for online dating adoption vs non-adoption, *Internet Research*, 31(1): 341–75.

Couch, D. and Liamputtong, P. (2008) Online dating and mating: the use of the internet to meet sexual partners, *Qualitative Health Research*, 18(2): 268–79.

Couch, D., Liamputtong, P. and Pitts, M. (2011) Online daters and the use of technology for surveillance and risk management, *International Journal of Emerging Technologies and Society*, 9(2): 116–34.

Department of Health (2020) *Social Work with Adults: Why Intersectionality Matters for Social Work Practice in Adult Services* [online], Available from: https://socialworkwithadults.blog.gov.uk/2020/01/31/why-intersectionality-matters-for-social-work-practice-in-adult-services/.

Earp, B.D. and Grunt-Mejer, K. (2021) Robots and sexual ethics, *Journal of Medical Ethics*, 47: 1.

English, B. and Tickle, A. (2018) Views and experiences of people with intellectual disabilities regarding intimate relationships: a qualitative meta-synthesis, *Sex and Disability*, 36(2): 149–73.

European Platform Sexual Assistance (EPSEAS) (2021) Vision and goals [online], Available from: epseas.eu.

Erens, B., Mitchell, K.R., Gibson, L., Datta, J., Lewis, R., Field, N. and Wellings, K. (2019) Health status, sexual activity and satisfaction among older people in Britain: a mixed methods study, *PLoS ONE*, 14(3): e0213835.

Evans, D.S., McGuire, B.E., Healy, E. and Carley, S.N. (2009) Sexuality and personal relationships for people with an intellectual disability. Part II: staff and family carer perspectives, *Journal of Intellectual Disability Research*, 53(11): 913–21.

Everett, B., Young, J., Carlson, M. and Clements, G. (2010) New British Columbia guidelines for supporting sexual health and intimacy in care facilities, *Healthcare Management Forum*, 23(1): 21–4.

Fosch-Villaronga, E. and Poulsen, A. (2021) Sex robots in care: setting the stage for a discussion on the potential use of sexual robot technologies for persons with disabilities, in: *Companion of the 2021 the 2021 ACM/IEEE International Conference on Human-Robot Interaction* [online], Available from: https://dl.acm.org/doi/proceedings/10.1145/3434074

Freak-Poli, R. (2020) It's not age that prevents sexual activity later in life, *Australasian Journal of Ageing*, 39(Suppl. 1): 22–9.

Gersen, J.S. (2019) Sex lex machina: intimacy and artificial intelligence, *Columbia Law Review*, 119(7): 1793–810.

Geymonat, G.G. (2019) Disability rights meet sex workers' rights: the making of sexual assistance, *Europe, Sexuality Research and Social Policy*, 16: 214–26.

Gillen, S. and Reynolds, P. (2021a) Ageing, physical disability and desexualisation, in P. Simpson, P. Reynolds and T. Hafford-Letchfield (eds) *Desexualisation in Later Life: The Limits of Sex and Intimacy*, Bristol, pp 95–116.

Gillen, S. and Reynolds, P. (2021b) Ageing, intellectual disability and desexualisation, in P. Simpson, P. Reynolds and T. Hafford-Letchfield (eds) *Desexualisation in Later Life: The Limits of Sex and Intimacy*, Policy Press: Bristol, pp 117–34.

Gruskin, S., Yadav, V., Castellanos-Usigli, A., Khizanishvili, G. and Kismödi, E. (2019) Sexual health, sexual rights and sexual pleasure: meaningfully engaging the perfect triangle, *Sexual and Reproductive Health Matters*, 27(1): 29–40.

Hankivsky, O., Grace, D., Hunting, G., Giesbrecht, M., Fridkin, A., Rudrum, S., Ferlatte, O. and Clark, N. (2014) An intersectionality-based policy analysis framework: critical reflections on a methodology for advancing equity, *International Equity and Health*, 13: 119.

Hategan, A., Bourgeois, J., Parthasarathi U. and Ambrosini, D.L. (2016) Counseling geriatric patients about opportunity and risk when 'digital dating', *Current Psychiatry*, 15(7): 74–7.

Health and Social Care Act (2008) *Regulation 9* [online], Available from: http://www.legislation.gov.uk/ukdsi/2014/9780111117613/contents

Helen Anderson Associates (2021) *Person-centred Thinking Tool* [online], Available from: https://www.helensandersonassociates.com/person-centered-thinking-tools/.

Hill, E. (2014) *We'll Always Have Shady Pines: Surrogate Decision-Making Tools for Preserving Sexual Autonomy in Elderly Nursing Home Residents* [online], Available from: https://scholarship.law.wm.edu/wmjowl/vol20/iss2/7.

Horne, M., Youell, J., Brown, L., Brown-Wilson, C., Dickinson, T. and Simpson, P. (2022) Feasibility and acceptability of an education and training e-resource to support the sexuality, intimacy and relationship needs of older care home residents: a mixed methods study, *Age and Ageing*, 6: 51(10): afac221.

Humphries, D.L, Sodipo, M. and Jackson, S.D. (2023) The intersectionality-based policy analysis framework: demonstrating utility through application to the pre-vaccine U.S. COVID-19 policy response, *Frontiers in Public Health*, 11: 1040851.

Jahnsen, S. and Wagenaar, H. (eds) (2017) *Assessing Prostitution Policies in Europe*, Routledge.

Jecker, N.S. (2020) Nothing to be ashamed of: sex robots for older adults with disabilities, *Journal of Medical Ethics*, 47(8), DOI: 10.1136/medethics-2020-106645

Kismödi, E., Cottingham, J., Gruskin, S. and Miller, A.M. (2015) Advancing sexual health through human rights: the role of the law, *Global Public Health*, 10(2): 252–67.

Koumpis, A., and Gees, T. (2020) Sex with robots: a not-so-niche market for disabled and older persons, *Paladyn, Journal of Behavioral Robotics*, 11: 228–32.

Kulick, D. and Rydström, J. (2015) *Loneliness and Its Opposite: Sex, Disability, and the Ethics of Engagement*, Duke University Press.

Lamphere, R.D. and Pomykacz, C.R. (2022) Love and discrimination: inequalities in online dating relationships in T. Flockhart, A. Reiter, and M. Hassett (eds) *The Reproduction and Maintenance of Inequalities in Interpersonal Relationships*, IGI Global, pp 23–46.

Larsson, A.T., and Jönson, H. (2018) Ageism and the rights of older people, in L. Ayalon and C. Tesch- Romer (eds) *Contemporary Perspectives on Ageism*, Springer, pp 369–82.

Lee, D.M., Nazroo, J., O'Connor, D.B., Blake, M. and Pendleton, N. (2016) Sexual health and well-being among older men and women in England: findings from the English longitudinal study of ageing, *Archives of Sexual Behaviour*, 45(1): 133–44.

Lester, P.E., Kohen, I., Stefanacci, R.G. and Feuerman, M. (2016) Sex in nursing homes: a survey of nursing home policies governing sexual activity, *Journal of the American Medical Directors Association*, 17: 71–4.

Linton, K.F. and Williams, L.R. (2019) Sustaining an intimate and sexually fulfilled marriage or partnership in older adulthood with a disability: perspectives of social workers, *Journal of Human Behavior in the Social Environment*, 29(8): 1026–35.

Malta, S. (2007) Love actually! Older adults and their romantic internet relationships, *Australian Journal of Emerging Technologies & Society*, 5(2): 84–102.

McAuliffe, L., Fetherstonhaugh, D. and Bauer, M. (2020) Sexuality and sexual health: policy in Australian residential aged care, *Australasian Journal of Ageing*, 39(Suppl. 1): 59–64.

Nwanazia, C. (2018) Sex care in the Netherlands – helping the disabled find intimacy, Dutch Review [online], Available from: https://dutchreview.com/culture/relationships/sex-care-in-the-netherlands-helping-the-disabled-find-intimacy/

Rahn, A., Jones, T., Bennett, C. and Lykins, A. (2020) Baby boomers' attitudes to maintaining sexual and intimate relationships in long-term care, *Australasian Journal of Ageing*, 39(Suppl. 1): 49–58.

Richardson, D. (2000) Constructing sexual citizenship: theorizing sexual rights, *Critical Social Policy*, 20(1): 105–35.

Richardson, K. (2015) The asymmetrical 'relationship': parallels between prostitution and the development of sex robots, *SIGCAS Computers & Society*, 45(3): 290–3.

Richardson, L.D. (2016) Integrating health equity into practice and policy, *Journal of Public Health Management Practice*, 22: S107–9.

Roelofs, T.S.M., Luijkx, K.G. and Embregts, P.J.C.M. (2021) Love, intimacy and sexuality in residential dementia care: a client perspective, *Clinical Gerontologist*, 44(3): 288–98.

Schwendel, G. (2020) *Joseph Rowntree Foundation: UK Poverty 2019/20: Social Security* [online], Available from: https://www.jrf.org.uk/social-security/uk-poverty-2019-20-social-security#:~:text=Three%20in%20ten%20of%20the,has%20persisted%20over%20recent%20years.

Shakespeare, T. (1996) Disability, identity and difference, in C. Barnes and G. Mercer (eds) *Exploring the Divide*, The Disability Press, pp 94–113.

Shapiro, L. (2017) The disabled sexual surrogate, *Reproductive Health Matters*, 25(50): 134–7.

Skills for Care (2020) *Supporting People who Need Care and Support to Have Meaningful and Safe Relationships* [online], Available from: https://www.skillsforcare.org.uk/resources/documents/Developing-your-workforce/Care-topics/Learning-disability/Supporting-meaningful-relationships.pdf.

Statista (2024) *Online Dating in the United Kingdom: Statistics and Facts* [online], Available from: https://www.statista.com/topics/12315/online-dating-in-the-united-kingdom/.

Taylor, B. and Davis, S. (2007) The extended PLISSIT model for addressing the sexual wellbeing of individuals with an acquired disability or chronic illness, *Sexuality and Disability*, 25(3): 135–9.

The Hebrew Home at Riverdale (2017) *Policies and Procedures Concerning Sexual Expression at the Hebrew Home at Riverdale*, RiverSpringLiving [online], Available from: https://www.riverspringliving.org/wp-content/uploads/2023/01/Resident-Sexual-Expression-Policy-revised-4.2017.pdf

The Royal College of Nursing (2022) *Older People in Care Homes: Sex, Sexuality and Intimate Relationships: An RCN discussion and guidance document for the nursing workforce* (3rd edn) [online], Available from: https://www.rcn.org.uk/-/media/Royal-College-Of-Nursing/Documents/Publications/2022/September/010-111.pdf

TLC Trust (2021) *Responsible Sexual Services for Disabled People* [online], Available from: https://tlc-trust.org.uk.

Touching Base (2021) *Sex Workers and People with Disability Coming Together* [online], Available from: https://www.touchingbase.org.

United Nations (2022) *Gender, Age and Disability: Addressing the Intersections* [online], Available from: https://www.unwomen.org/sites/default/files/2022-06/Brief-Gender-age-and-disability-en.pdf.

Vancouver Coastal Health Authority (2013) *Supporting Sexual Health and Intimacy in Care Facilities: A Pocket Reference Guide* [online], Available from: https://www.vch.ca/sites/default/files/import/documents/Supporting-sexual-health-pocket-guide.pdf

Villar, F. (2019) Sexual expression and sexual practices in long-term residential facilities for older people, in A. King, K. Almack and R. Jones (eds) *Intersections of Ageing, Gender and Sexualities: Multidisciplinary international perspective*, Policy Press, pp 153–70.

Villar, F., Celdrán, M., Fabà, J. and Serrat, R. (2017) Staff members' perceived training needs regarding sexuality in residential aged care facilities, *Gerontology and Geriatrics Education*, DOI: 10.1080/02701960.2015.1127811

Walker, A. and Foster, L. (2006) Ageing and social class: an enduring relationship, in *The Futures of Old* Age, Sage, pp 44–53.

Watt, S., Sword, W. and Krueger, P. (2005) Implementation of a health care policy: an analysis of barriers and facilitators to practice change, *BMC Health Services Research*, 5(53), DOI: 10.1186/1472-6963-5-53.

Wotton, R. (2020) Paid sexual services for people with disability: exploring the range of modalities offered throughout the world, in R. Shuttleworth and L. Mona (eds) *The Routledge Handbook of Disability and Sexuality*, Routledge, pp 433–49.

11

Final reflections: themes and issues arising from the volume

Paul Simpson, Trish Hafford-Letchfield and Paul Reynolds

This volume has showcased a variety of work by emerging and established scholars (based in and/or writing about contexts across Europe, Australia, Canada, Israel and South America). As such, it has featured a mix of theoretical and theoretically-informed empirical work variously from within sociology, social gerontology and social psychology, and covering a range of theories that includes insights from structuralism, poststructuralism and feminism. While we tried to include contributions from the global South and East, we came up against the sad reality that work on ageing sexuality is concentrated in the academies of the West and the global North (see Simpson et al, 2024). However, it is hoped that a volume in this book series, *Later Life Sex and Intimacy in the Majority World*, represents a useful start in addressing this inequality and in theorising ageing sexualities in parts of the global South and East (Ghisyawan et al, 2024), which are commonly obscured by the West's self-preoccupation.

In various ways and to varying degrees, all contributions to the volume have addressed the intersecting influences that help make up later life sexualities. If earlier volumes in the book series have focused on tendencies towards desexualisation of various older people, this volume has focused more on age (as it enmeshes variously with gender, sexuality, class and disability), but with greater focus on agency or agentic possibilities (and various) ambivalences. This is visible in various claims to sexual citizenship, recognition, respect and equal rights, and exclusion and inequalities in relation to them, which are at play in various cultural arenas.

The volume has also addressed some of the challenges of resexualisation. Although the contents of the volume represent a range of contexts, including online experiences in the digital age, inevitably, we can only claim to have presented some key, illustrative examples rather than a comprehensive survey of accounts of resexualisation. Nevertheless, we hope that the volume provides considerable insight, flavour and critical reviews of the state of current scholarship on the subject of resexualisation in later life. We also hope that it will inspire ideas for further research, policy development and practices that support older people as sexual and/or intimate beings, should they choose.

To avoid a simple, pedestrian recap of key points in individual chapters, this concluding chapter presents a synthesis of broader themes and issues that the contributions point to, though, inevitably, at strategic junctures, we refer to individual authors. Subsequently, we move to discuss what this volume indicates about the state of scholarship in an emerging field of knowledge and how this suggests an agenda or incipient manifesto that encompasses research, policy and practice.

Overarching themes relating to the resexualisation of older people

While the book is organised into two main (commonly overlapping) themes, reading across the ten substantive chapters that make up this volume, several overarching themes/issues become discernible. These themes concern reclamation via an alternative optics that enable reaestheticisation of older body-selves, the value of spaces and communities of understanding in facilitating positive resexualisation, and issues of control, inclusion and exclusion in relation to later life sexual citizenship.

Unsurprisingly, threaded through the volume is a strong theme of reclamation, (against the grain and beyond the superficial), but which concerns a more holistic desirability of older body-selves who are also seen as desiring subjects. Within the first section on cultures, we can see how this status can be attributed to a radically new and emergent aesthetic. This entails ways of seeing, forged in newer spaces by older people who will have grown up in an era that questioned traditional sexual mores and fought for bodily autonomy in various ways and from different subject positions. (The sex-positive dimensions of the women's movement and the LGBTQ movement spring immediately to mind.) In certain respects, this newer aesthetic is strongly suggestive of the continuity and generativity of the ageing process (Villar et al, 2024), and where previous experience and intergenerational struggles are drawn on and converted into demands and practices (whether conscious or unconscious, collective or individualised) that index recognition and respect as valid sexual beings. Such embodied reclamations are suggestive of the 'resources of ageing', which equip subjects with abilities to understand culture and challenge attempts at oppression (Heaphy, 2007; Simpson, 2015). The resources of ageing can sometimes operate independently of social class, but they are, inevitably, influenced by age, and complexly enmeshed with the effects of class, gender, ethnicity and disability, inter alia.

Indeed, to talk of multiple influences on the capacity to mobilise an alternative aesthetic is to talk of inequality. We see in the chapter by Liat Ayalon and Ateret Gerwitz-Meydan the effects of gendered patterns of use of online resources concerning various sex-related matters. In addition to drawing attention to new opportunities for resexualisation (through pharmaculture, 'bear' and silver daddy cultures and some D-I-Y pornographic narratives), Feliciano Villar and Ricardo Iacub, crucially add nuance to their analysis of resesexualisation in attending to age and gender inequalities, ambivalences and limitations that are attached to it. Their chapter provides a salutary reminder that while resexualisation is a worthy goal, not all forms of it are necessarily empowering, uplifting or challenging of the status quo. As we see in Barbara Marshall's chapter, one can be resexualised by other discourses and structures beyond one's control and in ways that are unwelcome. This means that there is still a huge amount of cultural labour to be done before older people are genuinely included (beyond fetishisation) in the sexual imaginary. Interestingly, Feliciano Villar and Ricardo Iacub have observed that opportunity for autonomous resexualisation exists currently more on the periphery of several cultures, pertaining to gay men and D-I-Y porn cultures. But, this applies much less to intergenerational heterosexual relationships and especially for old heterosexual women who 'fail' to embody the (ageist and sexist) capacity to look good or sexy 'for their age'. This may be less a 'failure' of the individual and more an inevitable failure of punitive, neoliberal, classist, sexist and ableist 'successful ageing' discourse.

Alternative sexual and relational aesthetics are also visible in chapters in the same section of the volume that address filmic representations. Most (but not all) mainstream media representations of later life sexualities tend to reinforce narratives of decrepitude, loss and disgust (sometimes in putatively comic mode) and, simultaneously, the dominant motif of desexualisation. Even so-called exceptions to this, like the film *Cocoon* (1985), tend to validate older people insofar as they are capable of mimicking youth. However, we can see how some films created within the independent sector are crucial in challenging and reversing such ageist discourses. Such moves are visible in the chapters by Eir-Anne Edgar (which also addresses non-monogamous representations on film) and by Paul Simpson and Megan Todd (addressing filmic representations of older lesbian-identified women and gay men). Both chapters analyse the film *Gerontophilia*, (2014) for its exploration of a cross-generational, inter-ethnic gay relationship that also operates as a (counter-intuitive) 'road movie'. Such alternative representations are indicative of a diversity of relational possibilities. They point to modes of relating beyond conventional representations of later life sex and intimacy that are commonly white heteronormative, cisgendered, monogamous and involve affluent/middle-class characters. Indeed, the films analysed either critically challenge fetishisation of older bodies while indicating to older *and* younger people, a form of aesthetics and practices that transcend the conventional misery narrative of inevitable decline into unsexiness, undesirability and ugliness.

Further, both of these chapters indicate how re-aestheticisation, resexualisation and a broader self-reclamation are dependent on a more critical optics. These ways of seeing entertain older subjects as 'watchable selves' by self and by others (Woodward, 2006) and are thus worthy of the erotic gaze. They also depict a more convivial humour around age and sexuality but working in more egalitarian mode *and* in spaces or relational configurations that are co-inhabited by others who are able to hear one's pain and joy. As Simpson and Todd conclude that, more critical representations, like those featured in the films discussed, have the power to dismantle the putatively stable ontology of who counts as sexy body age-wise and of who is allowed to desire whom.

Issues concerning convivial spaces and sexual autonomy are also taken up in the discussion by Nathalie Huitema-Nuijens and Tineke Roelofs, which addresses the resexualisation of disabled, older, long-term care residents in the Netherlands with the aid of dedicated sex workers. It should be recalled that disability correlates highly with age and that, globally, most disabilities are developmental (United Nations, 2023). Resexualisation through such means resembles a kind of non-medicalised healthcare (which, itself, promotes sexual health as part of holistic well-being) where the older disabled person is central to and drives decision-making. The enabling healthcare environments described in this chapter are predicated on and imbued with the humanistic principles of person-centred care. Some may be tempted to argue that, in a neoliberal age, person-centred care has become tokenistic or a hollowed-out cliché, adrift from the brute reality of a shrunken state where most care is self-funded (from sales of older people's homes and life savings).

However, this chapter, while showing the vitality of a continued sex/intimate life, provides a salutary reminder of the critical-humanistic thinking (against the grain of ageist erotophobia) in care organisations and systems and the collective consciousness and commonly observed policies and practices that are pre-requisite for resexualisation in care homes accommodating diverse older people. In the contexts the authors discuss, sex and intimacy seem to be normalised and are seen as a basic human need and right (though subject to careful negotiation). Unfortunately, here, too, we get a glimpse of neoliberal class inequality that imposes practical limits on who can afford sexual services generally and the more bespoke ones in particular. Similar themes are implicit in the final substantive chapter by Susan Gillen and Paul Reynolds on older disabled people and resexualisation, but which addresses a range of policies, practices and technologies and the various human, ethical and practical challenges they present. What stands out in their analysis is the call for a new way of regarding older disabled people, which encourages appreciation of them as socio-sexual citizens in ways that transcend their status as mere recipients of sexual services, aids and technologies, no matter how benevolent or well-intentioned. Of course, such thinking also reconnects us with the new aesthetic that invites us to think of older (disabled) people as part of the broader sexual imaginary.

Bridging the themes of culture with technologies and practices, Barbara Marshall's chapter raises important issues of macro-level relations of power and issues of control over resexualisation. In so doing, she offers another reminder, (though from a different angle), of the dangers involved in attempts at prolonging sexualisation and in resexualisation, past and present, which are currently tied to what can be a disciplinary discourse of 'successful ageing'. In light of this standard, one is obliged to wonder about those without the resources to embody this desired status or benchmark of older citizenship.

Furthermore, Barbara Marshall's chapter has usefully focused on the risks, inequalities and exclusions resulting from the ongoing medicalisation and 'pharmaceuticalisation' of sex in later life that reflect vested interests of the sexuo-pharmaceutiacal industry. The industry perpetuates not only (often older men's) anxieties over continuing sexual performance, but also reinforces narrow understandings of what counts as sex and who counts as an older sexual subject. As well as extending pleasure, resexualisation through pharma-technologies can also reduce sex in later life to a genitocentric, penetrative, reproductivist, ageist and heteronormative standard. We might therefore ask where do those thought to embody non-normative forms of gender and sexuality (and intimacy) fit into, if at all, such an agenda? This narrow focus also marginalises other forms of sexual, erotic and intimate enjoyment where the body might represent a whole field of possibilities, (which is more common in BDSM cultures). Such creative thinking is evident in accounts of participants (who tended to be culturally middle-class) in Simpson's (2015) study of middle-aged gay men in Manchester who reconceived sex beyond genitocentrism and youth- and orgasm-oriented penetration. In doing so, they questioned the very ontology of erectile dysfunction and penetrative sex (with its unequal notions of 'active' and 'passive' partners) as the gold-standard. Besides, Barbara Marshall's chapter also usefully points to an emerging body of academic work and a range of culturally-situated understandings of biological change that are critical of imperatives associated with sexuo-pharmaceuticals, which, in turn, form part of broader, disciplinary discourses of 'successful ageing' that reinforce inequalities in later life sexual citizenship. As counterpoint to this critique, the chapter also offers the beginnings of a manifesto for more positive, egalitarian forms of resexualisation, which we sketch further towards the end of this chapter.

Also bridging between culture and technology, and invoking themes of reclamation and (digital) spaces of opportunity, inequality and exclusions from resexualisation, the chapter on older heterosexual online dating by Christine Beasley and Mary Holmes observes the 'socially innovative' character of their accounts of practice that can defy the heteronormative standard. Interestingly, the chapter observes limits to the analytic utility of the concepts of gendered heteronormativity and ageist erotophobia. The varied, complex accounts of the more heterodox, older online daters mark limits to both concepts, indicating how older men (not hidebound by erection-anxiety) can feel comfortable about engaging in more mutual, egalitarian intimacies (associated with femininity) as a source of freedom from normally approved (youth-coded) masculinities. Conversely, we can see how some older women use internet dating for satisfying 'casual' sexual encounters (more associated with youthful masculinity). Such attempts at resexualisation, which can be complexly mixed with other, broader concerns about self-development and more avant-garde, platonic intimacies, destabilise notions of what 'proper relationships' should be. The chapter, then, offers a useful reminder that sex and intimacy enmesh with all manner of other issues and experiences concerned with power and esteem.

The same authors push their theoretical innovation even further in recalling that the creative subversions of older heterosexual online daters (when freed from genitocentrism) and their pushback against ageism are a timely reminder of the importance of changes wrought more gradually through smaller acts at a local level (rather than macro-level, grand narratives of revolution and rebellion). Indeed, Christine Beasley and Mary Holmes describe change and challenge to conventionality via a 'micro-politics.' This concept is redolent of Nikolas Rose's 'politics of the minor' which are, 'pragmatic, experimental … tentative … concerned with the here and now … the everyday not the transcendental' and which seek to bring about 'a small reworking of their own spaces of action' (1999: 279–80). Whatever the case, such accounts index a bodily confidence and autonomy that defy biomedical and popular discourses of loss and decline and upend stereotypes of desexualisation and the constraints of 'age-appropriate', demure femininity. Post-menopasual (or post-andropausal) is not post-sexual.

What joins the chapters in this text is the critical lens focused on the possible subversive spaces for resexualisation in social and particularly health contexts. This includes reclamations in representational practices and aesthetics and their bleeding into mainstream culture, and in the careful deployment of medical and technological supports as enabling, without accepting their deployment as simply managing deficit. Reynolds' discussion of kink offers a paradigm example of both the liberating possibilities of sex and intimacy beyond stereotypical genitocentric, gendered and `intimate' limitations that might enable some older people. At the same time, it can revert to some of the gendered power relations, social and cultural inequalities and patterns of exploitation that are characteristic of contemporary heteronormativity. This both underlines the value of different sexual sub-cultures, but also the need to accompany resexualisation with enabling choice and encouraging care, respect and communication in sexual relations.

Where now: research and the beginnings of a manifesto?

The themes underpinning this volume – of reclamation via alternative aesthetics, enabling spaces and communities of understanding, and power asymmetries relating to control and inclusion/exclusion – have prompted us to think about where to go in terms of research, policy and practice.

In terms of a research agenda, we would recommend further empirical research (and where possible, participatory methods involving co-production) that encourage wider dissemination of alternative aesthetics in portrayals of diverse older people across a range of media (old and new) and which represent them as valid sexual citizens. This intellectual project could be crucial in challenging stereotypes of automatic desexualisation and exploring further how various cultural spaces can become more inclusive of older people as legitimate sexual beings. This would, additionally, involve creative thinking about and authentic commitment to the resourcing needed to include those lacking the economic and cultural means to negotiate and flourish within such spaces.

A decent research agenda was also set out in the previous chapter by Susan Gillen and Paul Reynolds who recommended more studies on 'sex care' and appropriate technologies, and on policies and practices that enable sexual expression via information, products and services, and staff development in sexual health, aided by assessment and decision-making tools.

It is also worth reconsidering the idea, flagged in the chapter by Nathalie Huitema and Tineke Roelofs, of non-medicalised forms of health care that place the older (disabled) person at the forefront of decision-making about socio-sexual experience, strongly recommends itself. There are signs that such practices are beginning to take root and develop or, at least, warrant serious discussion. However, this would be dependent on a critical humanism becoming embedded and collectively observed in and across healthcare systems and organisations. By critical humanism, we refer to thinking beyond commonsense that centres equality, human needs, concerns and autonomy and regards such needs as outcomes of diversity and complex power relations.

In broader terms, a manifesto of sorts is available in Barbara Marshall's chapter where she cites Gupta (2019: 75) who 'suggests challenging a host of cultural assumptions around sexuality, gender and race' but could encompass: challenging the over-association of health and happiness with sexual activity (as part of punitive 'successful ageing' discourse); expanding sexual pleasure and fulfilment beyond genitally-focused, penetrative sex; critique of and looking wider than conventional 'scripts' of masculinity, femininity and heteronormativity; critique of sexual difficulties as largely biological and prioritise non-biomedical approaches (like sex education and counselling) as response to any such difficulties.

These recommendations variously urge getting several related issues into critical perspective. First, this involves thinking of sex as not the only/main source of contentment (or unhappiness) and that sex exists as part of a range of human experiences that can stimulate, satisfy and help promote overall well-being. Second, this project involves a similar critical intellectual and moral stance concerning ageist, reproductivist penetrative sex as 'the ultimate' (as commonly referred to heterosexual dating adverts) and of rigidified, gendered expectations of how older people should express their sexuality. Third, it is important that we recognise a plethora of non-medical 'solutions' to address sexual and emotional issues and challenges in later life.

Finally, while this volume has provided some rich insights into the many pleasures, dangers and ambivalences attached to the resexualisation of older people across a range of contexts, it is but a modest beginning in what is, inevitably, a long-term cultural-political project where much work remains to be done. But, we can, should and need to work towards the normalisation of diverse, complexly enmeshed ageing sexualities using both avant-garde, revolutionary and everyday micro-political means.

References

Texts

Ghisyawan, K., Harley, D., Shah, S. and Simpson, P. (2024) *Later Life Sex and Intimacy in the Majority World*, Policy Press.

Heaphy, B. (2007) Sexuality, gender and ageing: resources and social change, *Current Sociology*, 55(2): 193–210.

Rose, N. (1999) *Powers of Freedom: Reframing Political Thought*, Cambridge University Press.

Simpson, P. (2015) *Middle-aged Gay Men and Ageing: Over the Rainbow?* Palgrave Macmillan.

Simpson, P., Ghisyawan, K., Harley, D. and Shah, S. (2024) Introduction to the volume: themes, issues and chapter synopses, in K. Ghisyawan, D. Harley, S. Shah and P. Simpson (eds), *Later Life Sex and Intimacy in the Majority World*, Policy Press, pp 1–18.

United Nations (2023) *Disability* (Factsheet), United Nations.

Villar, F., Lawford, H.L. and Pratt, M.W. (eds) (2024) *The Development of Generativity across Adulthood*, Oxford University Press.

Woodward, K. (2006) Performing age, performing gender, *National Women's Studies Association (NWSA) Journal*, 18(1): 162–86.

Filmography

Cocoon (1985) Ron Howard, USA: 20th Century Studios.

Gerontophilia (2014) Bruce La Bruce, Canada: Film Option International.

Index

References to figures appear in *italic* type; those in **bold** type refer to tables.

T

U

V

W

X

Y

Z